ATHLETE AT HEART

Learning to live with heart disease and find joy again

KRISTINA BANGMA

Athlete at Heart

by Kristina Bangma

Copyright © 2023

First Edition

E-book ISBN: 978-1-7389889-1-4

Softcover ISBN: 978-1-7389889-0-7

All rights reserved. No part of this book may be used or reproduced in any manner without written permission, except in the case of brief quotations.

Editor: Elise Volkman
Cover Illustration: Jeremy Kersey
Cover Text & Interior: Kristy Twellmann Hill
Author Photography: Kevin Clark Studios

To Facundo and Naiya;
always forward, never back.

CONTENTS

	Introduction	1
1.	Someone Call 911	5
2.	How I Got Here	17
3.	It Takes More Than That to Scare Me	27
4.	Oblivious of the Consequences	39
5.	Next of Kin	47
6.	Plumbers and Electricians	53
7.	Animal in a Zoo	57
8.	Diagnosis Denial	65
9.	Living in a Beta-Blocker Fog	73
10.	Plan A	79
11.	Is It Worth the Risk?	85
12.	Breaking Point	97
13.	First Step Forward	107
14.	No Sick Days	113
15.	Bras and Marathons	119
16.	Sticky Cups of Gatorade	125
17.	A Matter of Perspective	129
18.	What If This Works?!	137
19.	Wedding Bells	143
20.	Getting Curious	149
21.	My New Super Power	157
22.	Cheater	165
23.	We Did It!	173
24.	Into the Canyon	179
25.	Return to Cypress	191
	Afterword	197
	Bibliography	203
	Acknowledgements	205

INTRODUCTION

The doctor warned me that I could die if I continued to exercise. I didn't believe him. I was an endurance athlete, performance triathlon coach, cycling coach, and personal trainer. I built my business on the belief that exercise was the key to good health and longevity, and I couldn't imagine my life without it. For a year, I lived in denial, testing my mortality. I played Russian roulette with every bike ride and training workout. I was determined to find a cure where there wasn't one.

Arrhythmogenic right ventricular cardiomyopathy (ARVC) is a rare, genetic, progressive heart disease and one of the leading causes of sudden death among athletes. Many are diagnosed only after an autopsy, and I know of others who have had near-death experiences. I am one of the lucky ones. I was warned, had plenty of time to prevent a cardiac arrest, and was fortunate to live in Canada where medical care is universal and, therefore, free. Not having to choose between what I could financially afford and what I needed likely saved my life.

When my heart could no longer keep up, I finally had to accept my fate and quit sports. I lost my identity as an athlete and questioned my coaching capabilities. All those hours that used to be dedicated to training were now spent contemplating my life's purpose. Continuing to teach and coach, but not being able to participate, was excruciating. Every day was a reminder of everything I had lost.

My journey wasn't easy, nor was it as linear as I have written it for this story. Any forced change is painful, but that is the purpose of suffering: to make our minds, muscles, bones, and hearts grow stronger (unless, of course, your heart is damaged, like mine). Although pain is inevitable and — when it comes to training your body — sometimes even desirable, we always have the choice of how long we are willing to suffer. Training for endurance sports taught me how to train my body. Living with heart disease taught me how to train my mind.

Every one of us will struggle with something in our lifetime. It could be injury, retirement, divorce, the death of a loved one, or losing a job, but nobody is immune. When it happens, we can choose to pivot and change, or stay the same and continue to suffer.

I made a promise to myself that once I learned how to live with my diagnosis, I would write about my journey to help others. During my search for answers, I couldn't find a book I related to as an athlete. Initially, I wanted someone to outline a step-by-step process for how to continue living when the one thing you loved most was taken from you. Now, having gone through the experience, I realize we have to find happiness in our own messy way. And so, although I am a personal trainer and coach who provides advice on all aspects of health and fitness, this memoir is not a self-help book or training guide for anyone diagnosed with heart disease. As best as I can recall, this is my story of acceptance, perseverance, personal discovery, and growth; along with my fears, misbeliefs, mistakes, and false starts. It is my hope that it will inspire you and maybe spark some ideas that you can use. My story revolves around endurance sports, specifically cycling, but I believe anyone looking to make a change can relate. Nobody can take away the pain of your struggle, but hopefully you can take comfort in knowing that you are not alone.

I was diagnosed with ARVC in 2016; therefore, many of my experiences are unique to the timing and the available research of that time. Medications, procedures, and exercise recommendations for heart arrhythmias have evolved since then, and continue to do so every year.

I am forever grateful to the team of doctors and nurses at the BC Inherited Arrhythmia Program (BCIAP) for all of their efforts in keeping me alive, especially in the beginning, when I was naive and ignorant of the risks I was taking. All of the names in this book are real, with one exception which has been noted. My experiences and conversations are recorded as I remember them happening; however, as is true in every conversation, what I heard (especially when speaking to anyone in the medical field) is only what I was capable of hearing at that time. What I left with, how I interpreted their words, and how they made me feel, may not have been what was intended, or I may have remembered only the worst of it. No two people will ever remember the same event in the same way, so I have done my best to share my journey as truthfully as possible, from my vantage point at the time. Every one of the doctors named has had a chance to read through a copy of this story and has granted me permission to use their real names and the conversations as they have been recorded.

I loved my life and everything about it before my diagnosis. But living through the struggle of having it all taken away has given my life a richness I had to learn to appreciate. There isn't a single day that I don't think about my heart disease. However, this daily reminder that my life is both precious and fleeting has made me grateful for each day. I am determined to make the most of my time on this earth.

CHAPTER 1

SOMEONE CALL 911

It was August 16th, 2015, the morning of the 8th annual Cypress Hill Challenge. A gentle breeze was barely noticeable as the sun began its slow creep across the sky — the perfect morning for a bike race.

I stood straddling my bike just behind the 40-minute marker. My boyfriend, Facundo, was ahead of me in the first wave, hoping to rival that day's fastest cyclists. Scattered throughout each of the time corrals were at least 30 Kits Energy riders, members of the cycling club I owned, among the 675 participants in the event. While waiting for the race to begin, I scanned the crowd for the Kits Energy black-and-white jerseys.

"Have a great ride!" I shouted to one cyclist, taking her photo. "See you at the top!" I said to another, giving him a high-five.

My hands were shaking with nerves, so after taking a few more group shots, I put my phone away. I spent the last few moments moving my attention away from the other riders and into my own race mindset. I needed to switch modes from being a coach to being an athlete.

When competing, I was nervous before every race. Sometimes the nerves were because I so badly wanted to win. Other times, I didn't have a chance of winning but was worried about crashing, which is always possible when riding a bike. But the main rush of adrenaline came from the realization that I must put myself through a severe amount of pain to achieve my best. Having the ability to embrace pain was essential to training and racing. Ignoring it wasn't enough — I had to welcome it. During training, I learned to anticipate the feelings that came with pushing myself to my limits; my heart beating loud and strong in my ears, my rib cage expanding, trying to accommodate more oxygen, and the familiar lactic-acid burn in my quads that made them feel like they were going to explode. Instead of resisting it, I reminded myself that the pain was temporary and, as much as it hurt, it would not damage me.

If I wasn't in pain during a hard training day or race, it meant that I had more to give. But once the pain arrived, I could finish without any regrets. The key was to ride that fine line of being on the edge of my limit without pushing beyond it, until the last few minutes. Learning where this line was came from training, experience, and strictly following my watt numbers.

Using a power meter helped me mitigate the error of going out too hard too soon. A power meter calculates the amount of power or force the rider produces second by second and is measured in watts. This information was transmitted and recorded by a small computer positioned on my handlebars. My computer was called a Garmin.

Although I always had butterflies in my stomach before a race, the moment the gun went off, all my nervousness evaporated and I entered into a state of bliss. I loved racing. I loved the feeling of concentrating on a single objective, where the only thing that mattered was crossing the finish line within the fastest time possible.

So I was relieved when the first two waves of riders had finally gone, and our turn came. With about 80 other riders in my time corral, I slowly followed the pace car, which controlled our speed until the start of the climb. As soon as the car pulled away, it signalled that the race had begun, and everyone picked up the pace. My nervous energy transformed into focused attention.

I felt both physically and mentally strong that morning and was excited to execute my plan. As I settled into my race pace, I glanced down at my Garmin and saw I was pushing 250 watts — 25 watts more than I had planned. I took a deep breath to calm myself and slowed back down to 225.

The watt numbers on the screen held immense power, to the point of even determining my feelings of self-worth as a rider and athlete. If I couldn't produce the same watts as I had in a previous race, event, or ride, I would berate myself and try to find out why. If I surpassed the expected numbers, I would proudly boast about it, posting it on Strava — an app for athletes — so all my riding friends, known and unknown, could marvel at my new personal record.

For the Cypress Hill Challenge, my self-worth was valued at 225 watts. If I could hold that number for the total distance of 12 kilometres, I would beat my fastest time of 40:53 from each of the previous 4 years.

While racing, I felt like I had two responsibilities to fulfill: perform as an athlete and be motivational as a coach. I recognized riders in my periphery, but kept my eyes focused on both the wheel in front of me and the watts on my Garmin, monitoring them simultaneously and religiously. I could not risk blowing up before the finish. Still, when I passed someone I knew, I offered words of encouragement.

"You got this! Way to go! See you at the top!"

I climbed the familiar mountain and continued to work my way from rider to rider. By the 9-kilometre mark, I was back to pushing 250 watts, but didn't slow down this time. With only 3 kilometres left before the finish, I knew I had it in me to hold the pace.

Excitedly, I yelled to my client, who had been riding with me, "We're at the last quarter mark. Now's the time to pick it up. Let's GO! GO! GO!"

Without any hesitation, he followed my command and surged, pulling ahead. I changed gears and attempted to jump on his wheel, but an invisible hand pulled me back. I watched with horror as the power on my screen dropped by half. I felt dizzy, out of breath, and slightly sick to my stomach.

Over the past two years, this had occurred more frequently when racing, so I didn't panic. It meant that I had crossed that fine line. All I had to do was slow down for a few seconds and let my heart rate lower; then, I could continue. Usually, in any other type of bike race, I could coast behind another rider or take advantage of a downhill, but when climbing a mountain, neither option was possible. I couldn't believe that I would actually have to stop.

Damn! I never, never stop in a race, not even to pee or eat! But I had no choice. This was unlike anything I had ever experienced. I had to bring my heart rate down or risk passing out and crashing on my bike.

But stopping didn't make me feel any better. My vision continued to narrow until the only thing I could see was the small patch of pavement immediately under my front wheel. Instinctively I knew I needed to lie down before I passed out. I unclipped from my pedals and laid my bike on its side just off the road. Without removing my helmet, I lowered myself down into the ditch beside my bike. The ground was overgrown with tall weeds and loose pebbles, but it felt soft and welcoming. My eyelids felt much too heavy to keep open. Drawing my knees close to my chest, I allowed myself to be lulled into the darkness.

Several riders stopped and hovered above me. I couldn't hear what they were saying but I no longer cared. Everything that had held such immense importance just moments earlier — the race, my watts, my clients, my boyfriend — none of that mattered anymore. I didn't even care that I was lying in the ditch in the middle of a bike race. At that moment, I only wanted to continue sliding into a blissful, peaceful state of nothingness.

Someone knelt close beside me in the ditch. A man's voice spoke loudly. His lips brushed my ear as he enunciated every syllable. Even so, the words felt like they were coming down a long tunnel from far away. He had so many questions.

"Did you fall? Do you have any chest pain? Are you on any medications?"

I whispered, "No. No… No."

I wanted him to go away or at least be quiet. But he persisted. My silence must have frightened him because his line of questioning became anxious and impatient.

"Tell me what's wrong! What do you feel?" he screamed at me.

With no emotion whatsoever, I answered, "Like I'm going to die."

It was true. Lying in the ditch, I felt no pain. I only felt as though my life was slipping away. I wasn't afraid, nor did I attempt to fight it. I simply lay there, waiting for whatever would happen next.

That one partial sentence propelled the man into action.

"Someone call an ambulance! Call an ambulance! An AMBULANCE!" He repeated the words a notch louder with each iteration.

For a second, I felt a thin glimmer of self-consciousness creep in. The idea of having my clients or even strangers witness me being rolled away on a stretcher because I couldn't handle one small mountain climb was an embarrassment I would avoid at almost any cost.

But then I relaxed back into my bed of weeds. An ambulance is usually on-site during a bike race, but Cypress Mountain had weak cell coverage. Someone would have to ride ahead to find cell reception or ride the last 3 kilometres to the top to alert the paramedics. By the time medical help arrived, they would be too late.

***

From where I lay in the ditch, I heard the man with so many annoying questions run along the road, his cycling shoes clicking on the pavement as he screamed for help.

Sound! I realized that my hearing had fully returned, and with it also came full self-consciousness. My vision returned next, and the dizziness and nausea were gone. I felt absolutely normal again. It didn't make any sense. I sat up and looked around me, shocked at the chaos I had created. Several riders had stopped to help me and were now milling around on the road. I climbed out of the ditch and walked back to the road. I was so ashamed that I couldn't look at any of the riders directly. I didn't even thank the man who had attempted to help me. Instead, I screamed at them collectively, "What are you doing? Get back on your bikes! This is a race!"

I picked up my bike, swung my leg over the top tube, clipped my shoe into the pedal, and pushed off. Several made weak attempts to stop me.

"The ambulance is coming."

"Don't go; you might be injured."

I ignored them. I wanted to get away from them and the scene as fast as possible. I wanted them to forget my face and the name of my business printed in bold letters on every piece of clothing I wore. I knew they would regret stopping to help me. They wouldn't be getting the finishing times they had hoped for.

I rode hard, brought my watts back up to 225, and quickly caught up to a group of riders who had probably seen me lying in the ditch moments earlier. I may have even passed the cyclists racing to the top to alert the ambulance. I rode with my eyes aimed straight ahead, trying to unsee all of them.

I finished with a time of 44:05.

After crossing the finish line, I tried to explain to my friends what had happened. "I had to lie down in a ditch halfway through my race."

They looked at me strangely and I realized how ridiculous it sounded. I found Facundo, but he was so excited about his own race that he wasn't listening to me.

"I finished in a time of 32:36, a few minutes behind the winners," he screamed over the loud music. He had executed a perfect race and was still on an endorphin high.

I turned to another friend. "The strangest thing happened today," I said. "I was having a great race and feeling really strong, when suddenly the world started closing in and I had to stop."

She brushed her hand in front of her face as though she were swatting away a fly. "Oh, you're probably just dehydrated. Why don't you get out of the sun?"

Nobody thought it strange that I'd felt the need to lie down in the middle of a race. I followed her advice and stood under a sponsor's tent, sipping Gatorade. Surrounding me, several other cyclists were talking about their races and complaining about how their event had been ruined.

"I would've had a good time, but had to stop for this drama queen."

"She said she was going to die and then got back on her bike and passed everyone as she raced to the top!"

"—this woman who was faking some sort of illness."

Nobody recognized that their so-called drama queen was standing right beside them.

I felt the need to explain myself, but what could I say? I wanted to stand on the podium and yell through the megaphone so everyone could hear that I had honestly felt like I was going to die. But there I was, feeling fine. They were right. They did stop for nothing, and now the damage was done, and their race was ruined. They wouldn't be able to brag to their friends or post this race on Strava. Instead, they would go away with a story about a woman wearing a Kits Energy jersey who had decided to stop in the middle of the race and make a scene, claiming she was dying. The implications of what I had done were irreversible.

I left the tent and walked back to the finish line, wanting to surround myself with people who didn't yet know about my fainting spell. Cheering on my club riders, I took their photos as they crossed the line. After they had recovered and unclipped from their pedals, I gave each of them a congratulatory hug and listened to their race stories.

When they asked about my race I told them, "Oh, I wasn't having a good day."

I wanted to explain why I was so much slower than previous years, but I couldn't think of a good excuse, nor was I going to confess that I had to stop to rest. I knew they would look up my time online when they got home. That's what endurance athletes do — especially recreational athletes. Since we aren't winning medals, we compete with each other and judge our success by comparing our times with friends and rivals.

Usually, I relished the post-race celebrations. It was my equivalent of a cocktail party — socializing, catching up with friends, maybe even recruiting a few new members to the club. But I wasn't up for celebrating or socializing that day. To fulfill my duties as a coach, I needed to stay until the end. But inside I was cringing with embarrassment and desperately wanted to hide. I didn't stay for the award ceremony.

After all my club members crossed the finish line, I said my goodbyes to a handful of friends, and Facundo and I descended the mountain alone. In an attempt to maintain Facundo's pace, I had to ride inches from his back wheel. Even then, I knew he rode just slow enough so I could keep up. It took all my effort to stay with him — almost as much effort as I had pushed on Cypress — and yet I experienced no traces of the feelings I'd had during the race. In single file, we made our way down the highway, across the Lion's Gate Bridge, through Stanley Park, over the Burrard Street Bridge, and finally back to our apartment in Kitsilano. As we rode the familiar route, my thoughts drifted back to the morning's events, trying to make sense of them.

Maybe I made it all up. How is it possible to recover so quickly?

By the time we carried our bikes up the stairs into our apartment, I had convinced myself that the entire incident had been a product of my own making. I felt my humiliation turn into panic. When a client bonks by pushing themselves too hard too soon in a race, we use it as a learning experience. But I should have known better.

Looking for reassurance, I asked Facundo, "What will people think of me? How can I coach others when I can't even coach myself?"

"You shouldn't worry about what other people think," he said.

CHAPTER 2

HOW I GOT HERE

I consider my childhood to be ordinary and average. My father was self-employed as a general contractor, while my mother stayed home to raise five children; two girls and three boys. Although I had very little to complain about, I was not a happy child. Lacking an outlet for my endless supply of energy, I felt frustrated and anxious most of the time.

If you asked me what I wanted to be when I grew up, I'm not sure what I would have said. I had never shown enough interest in anything for long enough to develop any level of skill or talent. Nor was there a single job that I wanted to learn, or dedicate myself to eight hours a day, five days a week. It all seemed so boring.

During early adolescence, like many teens, I was hypersensitive and self-conscious. My body lacked any telltale signs of turning into a woman and without a skill or talent to fall back on, I felt unremarkable and invisible. Wanting to make a change, I decided to focus on developing some sort of talent, and hopefully at the same time, change the way my body looked. I started with what was most familiar to me: running.

I was athletic but not an athlete. I did not play many team sports, take ballet lessons, or do gymnastics. I climbed trees, built forts, rode my bike to school, and swam in our backyard pool. So I'm unsure how I came up with my first walk/run program; a magazine likely, or it was possible that I didn't have a plan. I can't remember. Like most things in my life, when I decide I want something, I jump in with both feet and figure it out as I go. Before bed one night, I laid out the same clothes I usually wore to gym class — an old pair of cotton shorts, baggy tee shirt, and white sports socks. At 6 a.m. the following day, when my alarm went off, I jumped out of bed and was out the door. We lived on a country road on the outskirts of Peterborough, ON, so I had two options: right or left. Right had a small hill, so I chose left.

Running in the quiet early morning hours was calming. Besides the occasional car, all I heard were my white Asics running shoes hitting the gravel and my steady, rhythmic breathing. I loved feeling the power of my legs driving me forward and the sound of my heart pounding strong in my chest. As I returned home, I felt invigorated and energized. I also discovered that while running, the rest of the world melted away, and for just those few moments on the road, I was happy and felt calmer. The feeling slowly dissipated throughout the day, but the release of pent up energy was exactly what I needed. It didn't take long before I was addicted to running.

My older sister, Jan, warned me that habits were easily broken by missing just one day. I believe she was referring to the discipline of making my bed every morning. Still, I applied this advice to every habit I wanted to keep and would head out every morning. Soon, my 2-kilometre walk/jog turned into a daily 10-kilometre run. After returning from a run, I felt strong and powerful, like I could accomplish anything. Not only did I love the feeling of running, I relished the label of being a runner.

This was when I decided I wanted to be an athlete when I grew up (though outdoor enthusiast is probably more accurate). I didn't aspire to be a professional athlete. I simply wanted to be good at everything — specifically anything that involved being in the mountains. In my dreams, my future life would be filled with adventure and travel to exotic places, or anywhere outside of Ontario where there are no mountains.

However, I was still far from being the athlete I envisioned. My next goal was to become as strong as the boys. My older brother Paul and his friends taught me the basics of weight training and I started drinking protein shakes to "bulk up." At the very least, I wanted to look intimidating enough that anyone would second-guess messing with me. Being highly sensitive and extremely insecure, I was an easy target for teasing and bullying. The girls could smell it from a mile away and I thought that if I could look like someone who was physically strong, maybe I could pretend to be emotionally strong as well. Lifting weights wasn't as relaxing as running, but it released endorphins which made me feel invincible.

The next sport I truly fell in love with was road cycling. I spent every penny in my bank account (yes, we had pennies back then) on a red Trek 1500 road bike. I taught myself how to clip into the fancy pedals and rode that bike everywhere. After a year, when I thought I was a pretty accomplished rider, I joined the local bike shop's Saturday morning ride. I was the only female and the youngest rider by far. To me, all of the men looked ancient, but when you're 16, anyone over 30 looks old. So I was shocked when, in the first few kilometres of the ride, the old men dropped me like I was standing still. I pushed hard on the pedals and desperately tried to keep up, but I wasn't strong enough. My legs burned, my chest ached, and I could taste blood at the back of my throat. One man was kind enough to circle back and ride with me for the rest of the route, but I never went back. Not only was I mortified that I couldn't keep up with a bunch of old people, but I also didn't enjoy being in pain when exercising. I hadn't yet learned to appreciate and welcome it.

Thinking that I might be a better runner than cyclist, I joined our high school cross-country running team. At the sound of the gun, I shot off the line, leading the pack. I ran as hard as I could possibly go until I vomited my breakfast, and then limped the remaining distance to cross the line somewhere in the middle of the pack. You would think that after a few races I'd have learned my lesson, but my race strategy never varied. I didn't return the following year.

The only formal fitness training I received was during the three years I rowed in high school; likely the reason why I dreaded rowing practices so much. Rowing in that boat, petrified of "catching a crab," was the first time I willingly put my body through any intense pain to exercise. Catching a crab is a term rowers use to describe when you're out of sync with the boat. Your blade gets trapped in the water and, as the boat glides forward, the stuck blade will often fling the rower into the water. It is both painful and scary. But even with this fear and the realization that every practice and regatta would induce immense pain, I never quit. Enduring this pain brought me closer to becoming the athlete I wanted to be.

By grade ten, I was running 10 kilometres every morning before riding my bike to school, rowing practices, and my part-time job at Baskin Robbins. I hated that job, but scooping ice cream for a year paid for the training courses I needed to land my dream job as a lifeguard. On my 16th birthday, I secured my first lifeguard position at the YMCA, which came with an added perk of free access to the pool and weight training facility; a huge step up from the high-school gym.

My family and friends didn't understand my passion for exercise and teased me, which made me feel grossly misunderstood. Although I craved the camaraderie of others who had the same interests, it never deterred me from exercising. Since I didn't compete or compare myself with anyone, every workout felt like a win. I trained by feel, exercising for as long as it felt good and stopping when I was tired. I was rarely injured and always finished a workout feeling better than when I started. Without realizing it, I had created a well-balanced training plan and built a solid fitness base that would serve me well in my future years as an endurance athlete. Exercise provided a positive outlet for my endless energy, helped build my self-confidence, and 100% shaped my identity as an adult.

Post secondary, it seemed obvious that I would get a degree in kinesiology. I completed one year at the University of Waterloo, but the only future I could envision was an enormous debt in student loans and very limited job prospects. I needed to find a more economical path to achieving my dream life of living and working in the mountains.

I moved back into my parents' basement and registered for the hotel and resort management course at Fleming College close by. After my first year at Fleming, I took a job working at the Banff Springs Hotel in Banff, AB for the summer. I needed to finally discover if I really did enjoy living in the mountains for real, not just in my dreams.

Up to this point, I still didn't consider myself to be an outdoor athlete and was excited to begin developing this new part of my identity. So even though I was already in debt with student loans and I had never gone mountain biking before, I borrowed money from my brother-in-law Steve and bought my first mountain bike. With absolutely zero knowledge of what type of bike I would require for the trails in Banff, I chose a grey steel bike that was within my budget.

Within the first few weeks of living in Banff, I was crushed to discover that the athletes who I hoped would teach me how to ride and hike lived in Canmore, AB, which is a 20-minute drive from Banff. Without access to a vehicle I met only one cyclist that summer who offered to teach me some basic skills. After four depressing months of being so close to my dream life and unable to access it, I returned home with very little outdoor skills or experience. However, all was not lost. I had learned two valuable lessons: I didn't enjoy working in the hotel industry, but living in the mountains was exactly where I wanted to be. I was now willing to do whatever it took to get back there. I changed tactics and decided that I needed to acquire a skill that provided a flexible schedule and allowed me to travel and work anywhere. I quit hotel and resort management and moved to Toronto, ON to become a Registered Massage Therapist (RMT).

At 21, in the spring of 1998, and the day after I finished my RMT board exam, I moved from Toronto to Whistler, BC to start my dream life. I found friends who mentored me and shared my passion for outdoor sports. My new friends trained in a similar fashion, doing what they enjoyed for as long as it was fun. I didn't follow a formal training plan but continued to improve daily through repetition and learning from others. In the 90s, Whistler was still a seasonal resort, so I worked three jobs to maintain a steady income — massage therapist, lifeguard, and first-aid instructor. I worked hard and often double shifts, but I played harder. Seven days a week, I would ski, snowboard, hike, snowshoe, weight-train, cross-country ski, mountain bike, or swim in the lake. My life felt surreal and surpassed my wildest dreams for my future self. For three years, I felt like I had found heaven on earth.

But after too much repetition, even paradise can get boring. I needed a new challenge and relocated to Vancouver, BC. Having enjoyed a very comfortable and easy lifestyle, leaving the protective bubble of Whistler was difficult and disorienting. For the first few years in the city, I struggled and suffered from a few setbacks and tough breaks. But in 2003, I found my footing again and started my own personal training company.

Up until this point in my life, I had been obsessed with exercise because it felt good to be in motion and I always felt better after a workout. It wasn't until my 30s that I discovered racing and became addicted to the adrenaline rush of competition. In 2006, Chris, my boyfriend at the time, convinced me to race a 15-kilometre trail-running race in Squamish, BC called Loop the Lakes. When I crossed the finish line, Chris, who had already finished ahead of me, rushed towards me, yelling with excitement, "You won second! You won second place overall female!"

This surprised me. Compared to the athletes that I had trained with in Whistler, I was usually one of the slowest. Chris pumped me with compliments and encouraged me to start mountain racing with him. "If you trained a bit more, you could beat all the girls."

And he was right. For two years, it was often Chris and Kris on the podium, male and female. In my second season, I won first overall female of the 5 Peaks Trail Running series.

Once I got serious about trail running, I wanted to learn how to formally train for competitions. I bought a heart-rate monitor, read training books, and completed the certification courses to become a coach. But I didn't think that having knowledge was enough. I thought I needed to prove I could do it for myself before helping others achieve their goals. I pressured myself to become more competitive and designed a more rigid and disciplined training schedule. I exercised twice as hard as I had in Whistler. Not only did I follow my own training program, I also worked out with my clients in the gym, hiking Grouse Mountain, or pacing them in a running race.

Through trail running, I gained confidence that I could be a competitive endurance athlete. Within two years I was also training and racing in road running, road cycling, swimming, and eventually triathlon. Between all these sports I raced almost every weekend and every distance, including Ironman Canada in Penticton, BC. I was competitive in my age group and frequently placed in the top three.

I also obtained my certification as a triathlon coach and a certified performance cycling coach. I wanted to become an expert, a leader, and a coach in every sport I competed in. It was equally important that I maintained my status as a competitive athlete and also continued to grow as an endurance coach. Training, racing, and coaching had now merged into one entity, which I called my life.

I didn't have a master plan of where this racing and coaching would take me, but I was determined not to allow anything or anyone to slow me down. I didn't want anyone to distract me from this life I had created. Even socializing included some form of exercise, or at the very least, a walk. My first three dates with Facundo were all three-hour bike rides. If someone wanted to date me or be my friend, they had to keep up with me.

Facundo Chernikoff not only kept up but surpassed me in almost every sport. He is one of the few people I know who is unapologetically his own person, never downplaying his achievements but not bragging about them either. He is an old soul, more mature than his years, and an unconventional thinker who has the intelligence and ambition to solve almost any problem that comes his way. Being around him made me want to try harder and improve at everything I did. He was ambitious, but unlike me, he actually had a plan for his future.

Once we started dating, he helped me organize my company and my coaching business took off. It was a busy and hectic life; personal training, online coaching, running both a cycling club and running club, writing cycling and fitness articles for the Vancouver Courier and other various blogs, while also racing. I loved everything about it.

One sunny afternoon in July of 2013, in the middle of a workweek, I strolled the two blocks down from my apartment to the ocean for a swim workout. With my wetsuit half zipped up to the waist, I wore only my bathing suit, goggles, flip flops, and a towel thrown over my shoulder. When my toes hit the warm sand, I surveyed the beach, the people lounging in the sun, and the mountains standing proud on the North Shore. I laughed out loud in pure joy and some partial disbelief that this was truly my life. I had done it.

I never planned to retire. Why would I when I was having so much fun? I had worked through several broken bones and minor surgeries, which had made my job more complicated, but I always found ways to work around them. I expected that I would teach chair aerobics well into my 80s.

I never imagined that I would be diagnosed with a disease that forbade exercise and threatened to destroy everything I had worked my entire life to build.

CHAPTER 3

IT TAKES MORE THAN THAT TO SCARE ME

Fainting on the mountain wasn't enough to scare me into seeking medical attention. Neither I nor any of my friends thought that my temporary loss of consciousness in the middle of a bike race was anything to be concerned about. My arrhythmia was actually discovered due to a more debilitating problem at that time: severe bouts with vertigo.

The vertigo attacks had started in the spring of 2014, more than a year before the Cypress Mountain incident. The first time it happened, I was demonstrating a push-up. When I got up from the floor, the room started to spin around me. I was so off balance that I could barely walk and grabbed onto the wall to prevent myself from falling back down. I made it home that day with difficulty, and it took a few days before I could return to work.

Riding a bike or driving during a vertigo attack was impossible. The vertigo I experienced wasn't the same as being lightheaded or dizzy, nor the same as what I was experiencing when I raced. With vertigo, the room flips up and down, spins, and rotates randomly, even with my eyes closed. It felt like being on an amusement park ride without the fun factor.

Facundo's theory was that the vertigo was linked to overtraining, but I didn't want to take any advice that required reducing my level of exercise. I consulted my family doctor, Dr. Bregman, who diagnosed it as benign paroxysmal positional vertigo (BPPV). He explained that fine calcium crystals dislodge in the inner ear canal, which causes the brain to receive confusing messages about body position. I called them attacks because the symptoms arrived suddenly, varying in intensity and severity. Small attacks made me sick to my stomach and slightly dizzy. They would sometimes last for only a few hours or they could linger up to several months. Either way, I could still perform daily activities and even exercise. A severe attack forced me back to bed to wait it out, which could take up to 24 hours. I had hoped that it would eventually go away on its own. However, after several months of debilitating vertigo that often prevented me from working and training, I went back to see Dr. Bregman. He gave me a prescription to help with nausea and suggested I see a physiotherapist.

"They can perform something called an Epley maneuver, which helps put the crystals back into place," he said. "But if that doesn't work, you just have to wait it out and learn how to live with it."

I booked an appointment with a physiotherapist who was supposed to be "the best at the Epley Maneuver" and was highly recommended. She explained the procedure: "From a sitting position, I'm going to push your upper body down onto the bed as fast as possible. Your head will hang off this pillow at a 45-degree angle. If your eyes are oscillating in this position, it is confirmation that your crystals are displaced, and we're not dealing with something else. After a few seconds, we'll roll you onto one side and wait again. Finally, you will sit back up to see if the procedure worked."

I informed her that all of this movement would probably make me vomit, but I was willing to endure it if she could fix me. She placed a bucket at the end of the table and began the procedure. Over and over, she threw me down on the table, and each time, I felt my eyes bouncing like marbles looking for a place to land. I had arrived at the appointment feeling well enough to drive, but with each attempt, I felt worse and finally begged her to stop.

She assisted me off the table and into the waiting room, where I slumped in a chair, my head in my hands. Irritated with wasting my time, I vaguely wondered if my parking meter had expired. No way would I be able to move, let alone drive, until this new bout of vertigo had settled. The receptionist swiped my Visa for the $85 charge and left me alone to contemplate my situation. I sat for another half-hour before I felt stable enough to drive.

Over time, I learned which movements could bring on a new bout of vertigo or worsen it.

The rules were:

1. Do not sleep, rest, or demonstrate any exercises while lying on my left side for any amount of time.
2. Any movement from one position to another — rolling from my stomach to my back, the reverse, or the transition from lying down to standing — must be performed in slow stages, never quickly.
3. When lying on my back, I must prop my head up slightly, either with a pillow or my hands.
4. Under no circumstances can I look up or roll my head backward.

I learned to adapt to feeling slightly off balance much of the time, and I could even teach a fitness class and demonstrate exercises without anyone knowing about my condition. At the time of this writing, I still suffered from vertigo and adhered to these rules most of the time. Eventually, I will discover the key to eliminating the attacks almost completely, but that's for another chapter.

***

Throughout 2015, the vertigo symptoms were almost always with me at various levels of severity and intensity. So when I woke up the Monday morning after the Cypress Hill Challenge, and the vertigo was back in full force, I wasn't surprised. I gingerly swung my legs over the bed and allowed the room to settle. Holding onto the wall for support, I walked ever so slowly to the bathroom and splashed cold water onto my puffy eyes. And as I did every morning, I lectured myself in the mirror. "Kristina, you need to get more sleep."

Coaching until 8 p.m. and waking up at 4:30 a.m. didn't allow for more than six — maybe seven — hours of sleep each night. It wasn't enough to fully recover from my busy lifestyle.

When the dizziness reduced to a manageable spin, I picked up the pace, conscious of the time. I was nauseous and didn't feel like having breakfast, and really, who wants to eat at 4:30 a.m.? But I had to force myself. My next opportunity to eat wouldn't be for another seven hours, after I was finished training clients. I dropped two eggs into the water to boil and a slice of bread into the toaster. While waiting for my breakfast, I changed out of my pajamas and into the gym clothes I had laid out the night before: a tank top, sweater, leggings, and running shoes, all in black. I ate quickly, not tasting anything, and poured my coffee into a to-go mug.

My dog, Naiya, paced between me and the front door, anxious to go out for her morning walk. I adopted Naiya, a wheaten-cross, from the SPCA in 2010, when she was 10 months old. She looked like a soft plush toy, and so adorable that anyone who saw her couldn't help themselves but stop to pet her. But she also had an endless supply of energy and demanded an enormous amount of attention; two hours of daily strenuous exercise to keep her from getting into some sort of mischief. With the moon still bright in the sky, we walked warily, both of us on watch for skunks and raccoons — or any other stray animal that could delay my morning.

No matter the hour, the environment at the gym was always the same. If the bright overhead fluorescent lights didn't wake me up, the music pumping out the latest popular mix on repeat and at max volume would definitely do it.

I arrived at the gym at the same time as Phil Teal. Phil had thick grey hair, wore wire-rimmed glasses, and greeted everyone with a sweet, patient smile. I waited for him to lock his car and held the gym door open for him. Like many early-morning clients, Phil arrived wearing gym clothes and carrying his suit bag and a pair of dress shoes for work. This simple change of clothing would transform him from Phil into Dr. Teal, neurologist, and director of the Vancouver Stroke Program. As he was early for his training session, I took the time to ask for his advice on my vertigo.

"I'm really sorry, Kristina, but your doctor is correct," he answered. "The Epley maneuver is the only thing we're currently aware of that can dislodge the crystals."

I wasn't convinced. "How do people live with this? For over a year, I've been trying to manage it, but some days I can barely walk, let alone ride a bike or drive a car. How am I supposed to work, train, and race with a problem that's so unpredictable? I'm scheduled to race the 145-kilometre distance in the Victoria Fondo this weekend but I can't do that if I have vertigo."

"Well, the maneuver only works if you do it correctly," he said. "Come to my office on Thursday. I'll see if I can dislodge the crystals for you."

"Thank you, thank you, thank you," I gushed and restrained myself from giving him a huge bear hug.

On Thursday, I rode my single-speed bike the short distance to Vancouver General Hospital. I took my time locking my bike to the rack, ensuring that it was secured and hidden among the others. Vancouver was notorious for bike theft, so this was the only bike I would ever risk locking up outside. The bike itself was not expensive. The white paint was chipped, exposing the steel frame and the beginnings of rust, and the rims were mismatched, one black, one green. But I loved her just as I did all four of my bikes, and would be sad to lose her.

As I triple-checked the lock, I felt ashamed for having asked Dr. Teal for help. He dealt with cases much more severe than mine — actual life-and-death situations. His expertise shouldn't be wasted on minor inconveniences affecting a weekend bike race. But I couldn't back out now. Pushing my guilt aside, I stuffed my helmet into my backpack and marched into the hospital. My running shoes squeaked on the polished marble floors as I followed the directions to the neurology floor.

The receptionist greeted me with a smile. As she led me down the hall to the examining room, my guilt was replaced with anxiety. Doctors, even doctors I knew well, made me nervous. Maybe it was because they knew more about my body than I did, which made me feel vulnerable and insecure. Every time I sat in a doctor's examining room, I felt myself crumble to mush.

While training clients in the gym, I didn't think of them as doctors, lawyers, or CEOs of billion-dollar companies. They were all just regular people in sweaty tee shirts and stinky running shoes. There, I was the expert and the one in charge. But the moment I walked into Dr. Teal's office, he was no longer Phil, a man striving to complete one more pushup. He was Dr. Philip Teal, and he was the expert.

I sat down on the plastic chair, feeling small and embarrassed for wasting his time. I reminded myself that my career depended on me being healthy. I couldn't afford to lose income because of crystals becoming dislodged in my ear. I needed to be confident that I could rely on my body to perform for me. In all my 13 years of working as a personal trainer, I could count on one hand the number of times I had cancelled a session because I was sick.

I convinced myself that I had a right to be there.

After a few moments, Dr. Teal arrived. He didn't waste any time. "Kristina, we think we know what the issue is, but I don't like to assume anything, so let's go over your history before we begin."

I dutifully answered his questions with a bunch of nos.

"No, I don't have any medical issues in my family, past problems, or current health issues, but…" I paused, unsure if the information was relevant.

He looked up from his computer. "Anything you can tell me might help," he encouraged.

"Well, I don't think this has anything to do with my vertigo because this just happened recently, and my vertigo started a year ago, but…I passed out in a race on Cypress Mountain last Sunday."

Remembering that Dr. Teal was also Phil from the gym, I followed this up with several excuses for why I had bonked. I didn't want him to think that I was a lousy coach. In an attempt to sound nonchalant, I explained, "This has happened in races before, but this was the first time I had to stop. The sensations come on suddenly and then are gone just as fast — so quickly, in fact, that I was able to get back up again and finish the race."

He continued to type, not saying anything for a few moments, so I continued. "But that isn't the same as the vertigo I have now. They're two very different experiences. I don't think they're related."

Dr. Teal stopped typing and turned his body away from the computer to look at me. His voice remained gentle but earnest. "Kristina, a healthy athlete like you should not be passing out or fainting, not in the middle of a race or any other time. I want to send you for a 24-hour Holter monitor test to measure your heart activity and refer you to a cardiologist, just to check it out."

"Fine," I said, secretly hoping that, with all these tests, they might discover a solution to my vertigo.

He set up the requisition and then turned to me again and said, "Ok, now, let's get you on the table and try to fix those crystals so you can race this weekend."

This time the maneuver didn't make my vertigo worse, but it didn't make me feel better either. At best, I left feeling about the same as when I had arrived. Since this was manageable, I was relieved. I thanked Dr. Teal profusely for spending his valuable time on me and agreed to follow up with the cardiologist when I returned from my vacation in September. Whatever Phil thought was wrong with me would have to wait until the cycling season was over.

***

Three days later, I stood on the starting line of the Victoria Gran Fondo, ready to redeem myself after my embarrassment on Cypress. The vertigo had subsided substantially and I was feeling strong. Although a fondo or gran fondo event isn't supposed to be a race, most riders treat it as one. Even when the event doesn't offer prizes or medals, it has a start, a finish, and a timing chip; therefore, it is a competition.

When the gun went off, I went into race mode and slid my bike into the middle of a fast group. I was feeling confident and, mentally, I was ready to perform. But my body had other plans. Once we left the city centre and the pace picked up, the symptoms I had felt on Cypress Mountain returned. I was forced to slow down and pull out of the group. As I fell behind, my riding buddy, Glen, looked back to see if I was ok. I smiled and gave him a thumb's up, signalling him to go ahead without me. I rode the remainder of the 145-kilometre distance alone, hating every minute of it. I still finished in a reasonably good time, but I knew for sure now that something wasn't right.

The following month, in training, I discovered that I could manage the symptoms by maintaining a heart rate below 160 bpm. But keeping my heart rate that low also meant I couldn't sprint or be competitive. With only one event left in the cycling season, the 122-kilometre Whistler Gran Fondo, I decided to give up the idea of racing it. Instead I rode the event with a team of club members, supporting and helping them get their fastest times. It felt glorious to ride in an event without putting myself in severe pain, and for the first time ever, I was able to take in and enjoy the beautiful scenery.

Five days after the Whistler Fondo, Facundo and I packed our bags for Greece and Turkey to celebrate my fortieth birthday. Before I'd met Facundo, I had always used vacations as an opportunity to train even harder than at home. It was Facundo's idea to spend the entire three weeks with no formal exercise — nothing that would require a heart rate anywhere close to 160 bpm. Overtraining is common among endurance athletes and we felt confident that, after some rest, I would recover and the problem would sort itself out.

CHAPTER 4

OBLIVIOUS OF THE CONSEQUENCES

Our trip to Greece and Turkey was a magical three-week vacation. We toured churches and mosques, flew in a hot air balloon in Cappadocia, drank wine while watching the sunset, and explored the beaches of Santorini and Mykonos on beat-up, old ATVs.

I was still on a vacation high when I rode my bike to Vancouver General Hospital on Thursday, October 8th, 2015; this time for the 24-hour Holter monitor test. I barely had enough time to pick up one of the six-month-old gossip magazines in the waiting room before a nurse called my name. She wore blue hospital scrubs and running shoes and her hair was tied back into a loose ponytail. I followed her down the hall to the examining room. She introduced herself — I'll call her Julia — and, without looking up from her clipboard, began asking questions.

After confirming my full name, date of birth, and home address, she asked, "So why are you having this test?"

I didn't respond immediately. The question should have been easy enough, but I had difficulty coming up with a reason that made any medical sense. Except for Dr. Teal, nobody else seemed to think anything was wrong with me.

Finally, I settled on the basic facts. "When I push myself hard during exercise, I feel dizzy and faint."

Hearing myself saying it out loud, it sounded ridiculous. I imagined what Julia must be thinking: *Who doesn't get dizzy and lightheaded when they push hard during exercise?* But I had been racing long enough that I knew what I was experiencing wasn't normal.

To help justify my need for the test, I added, "And I passed out briefly in a bike race a few months ago and haven't been able to race or train hard since."

I was embarrassed and waited for her reaction and judgement. But Julia just nodded and asked me to remove my tee shirt so she could place the sticky pads and attach the wires. I peeled off my shirt and sat on the examining table in my sports bra.

She turned back towards me and exclaimed, "Wow, you're really fit!"

I smiled sheepishly and gave her my standard one-line response. "Thanks, I'm a personal trainer."

Julia didn't skip a beat and said, "I'm sure you're a great runner; you should join our women's soccer team. We're looking for another player and you would be perfect!"

I fixed my gaze on the wall just over her shoulder as my inner voice quickly flipped from embarrassment to mild annoyance. Julia was a nurse and I was her patient. I'd just told her I was here because I had a problem exercising. But I also knew she was only trying to be friendly and, in any other normal circumstances, I would have taken her persistence as a compliment. Who doesn't want to be handpicked for a sports team? So I did my best to remain polite, turning her down lightly.

"I haven't played soccer since elementary school," I responded.

But she didn't let up. "Oh, but you would fit right in! We train every Thursday night and play games on the weekends."

She said this as though knowing the schedule would convince me to join her team.

I responded more firmly this time. "I don't like team sports."

At this point in the conversation, I was seething with anger and frustration. I couldn't believe that I had to make excuses for this stranger when I just wanted to get my life back to normal.

Fortunately, placing the sticky pads on my chest didn't take long. Julia attached the electrodes and fit the monitor into a small pack I was instructed to wear in a belt at my waist. I worried I might have hurt her feelings, but she didn't seem upset by my rejection. Unfazed, Julia continued with her work, explaining what would happen next.

"For the next 24 hours, go about your day as you normally would, except don't shower with it on. Tomorrow at 5 p.m., turn off the machine using this switch and remove the sticky pads yourself." Pointing to the switch, she continued, "You have until 6 p.m. to drop off the device before the office closes for the Thanksgiving long weekend. Once they've reviewed the information, someone will call to schedule an appointment with a cardiologist, which may take a few weeks. Do you have any questions?"

I did not.

For the next 24 hours, I did everything I would do throughout a typical week — all in one day. I woke up at 4:30 a.m., trained clients in the gym, put myself through a strength workout, and took Naiya for a power walk in the woods. I saved the most intense effort for the last hour, so I could shower after I had removed the monitor. My plan was to recreate the symptoms on my bike trainer at home by doing a 20-minute functional threshold power (FTP) test. The FTP test is one of the most grueling workouts you can do on a bike trainer and the closest to a race situation. My goal was to hold the same power I'd held on Cypress at 225 watts, or more, for 20 minutes, or until I felt close to passing out.

During the winter months, Facundo and I set up our bikes on trainers inside our apartment, allowing us to continue riding year-round. We lived in a 1,000-square-foot two-bedroom and used our second bedroom as a multi-purpose room. On one wall hung two mountain bikes, one above the other. On the other wall was a couch with a pull-out bed for guests, and our shared desk sat against the third wall. From mid-October until mid-March, our two road bikes were set up side by side in the middle of the room, facing our desk and each of our large screen monitors. Sometimes we rode together, but most often we rode separately while the other worked. We only realized how strange this setup appeared when we had visitors. They couldn't help but laugh and comment, "This place looks like a bike shop!"

I dreaded doing the FTP test and kept procrastinating. It was late in the afternoon before I finally started my ride, which didn't leave much time before Facundo had to leave for his night shift. He worked for the Vancouver Fire Department and would be gone until the following morning. Although we didn't think recreating the symptoms was dangerous, we did have some trepidation and thought it wise that I wasn't alone when I attempted it.

Starting with an easy 20-minute warm-up, I mentally prepared myself for the pain I would endure during the FTP test. Nearing the end of the test, Facundo stood up from his computer to stand beside me, cheering me on. He looked down at my Garmin, and when he saw my power drop, he encouraged me to ride faster.

"Come on! You can do it!"

"You have more than that!"

"Push your watts back up!"

With only a few minutes left until the end of the test, he started to get more aggressive. "Kristina, stop wimping out!"

But I was tired and couldn't motivate myself to take on more pain. Even though my legs and lungs were screaming, begging me to stop, my heartbeat was strong and steady. I had no nausea, tunnel vision, or feelings of passing out. I finished the test without anything happening.

Facundo threw his hands up in frustration. "You're wasting my time! You said you feel sick and lightheaded every time you ride hard! How come you can't replicate that now?"

I didn't have an answer for him.

"Forget it," he said. "I have to go to work. You're on your own."

Neither of us knew that what I was attempting to do could be dangerous for me. At that time, all we knew was that when my heart rate went over 160 bpm, I felt like passing out, and if I wanted someone to fix it, they needed to see why that was happening. At this point, I had replicated the symptoms in two cycling events and several times during hard training workouts. Each time, nothing terrible happened and I had resumed riding shortly after it passed.

Just before Facundo left for work, he threw back a suggestion. "Why don't you try running up and down the stairs? Don't you also feel dizzy when you do that?" And with that, he was gone for the night.

He was right. I had complained about feeling faint when running up and down the stairs to do laundry. I checked my watch and saw that I still had enough time.

Jumping off the bike, I changed from my cycling shoes to running shoes. Together, Naiya and I tore up and down the four flights of stairs in my apartment building. She loved this game and never tired of it, but I didn't last very long. After only a few minutes, my legs and lungs were fatigued again, but my heart was still steady.

Now I was angry with myself as well. *Kristina, you can NOT bring back this monitor without showing them the symptoms that you're complaining about. They'll think it's all in your head!*

Then, a second voice chimed in. *Maybe it* is *all in your head...?*

I returned to the apartment, jammed on my cycling shoes again, and jumped back on the trainer. Moving the chain into the heaviest gear, I started to pound on the pedals, around and around, faster and faster. I didn't listen to music or look at my Garmin, my watts, or the time. I told myself I would ride as hard and fast as possible until I passed out. I would not let myself stop until that happened. The more it hurt, the sooner the pain would be over.

And it was. Within a few minutes, the walls began closing in around me. I pushed a bit longer to ensure the sensation wasn't my mind playing tricks on me. Only when I felt that I had barely a few seconds left before I would pass out did I get off the bike. I laid myself down in the fetal position to wait it out. After a minute or so the feelings dissipated and I felt normal again. I stood up and turned off the Holter monitor, carefully doing everything Julia had instructed. I didn't want to repeat the test any time soon.

I texted Facundo to let him know I had succeeded. He sent me a thumbs-up emoji, and I felt proud of myself for being able to reproduce the symptoms. I considered the event as simply collecting data. Beyond being excited to get some answers, I wasn't concerned or scared. I had no idea what I had just done.

CHAPTER 5

NEXT OF KIN

Saturday morning, the day after I dropped off the 24-hour Holter monitor, Facundo and I went mountain biking together for the first time. It was a beautiful, warm fall morning, the start of a long-holiday weekend, and I was looking forward to a few days full of activities and dinners with friends. Facundo had recently bought himself a mountain bike and I was going to show him the trails I had been riding for years. During the half-hour drive to Mount Seymour on the North Shore, we talked about everything except for the previous day's Holter test. In our minds, there wasn't much to discuss until I got the results back.

Although mountain biking was my favourite sport, I didn't go as often as I would have liked, and it had been several months since my last ride in the trails. I assumed that was why, partway through the ride, I found myself gasping for breath. I should have known better — Facundo was always faster than me in every sport. Each time I gained a bit of ground on the downhill, he would overtake me on the climbs, yelling, "On your left!" as he passed, picking his way up and over the slippery tree roots and small rock ledges.

I was pedalling up a long, technical climb that I had ridden dozens of times before when the trees began to close in around me. Similar to when I was riding up Cypress Mountain, it was like a switch had been flipped inside of me. All I could yell was, "Facundo!" before getting off my bike and once again lying down in the fetal position in the dirt.

Naiya bounded back down the trail towards me. I closed my eyes as she began licking my face. Facundo took a bit longer, slowly working his way back down the steep rocky incline. When I opened my eyes again, he was straddling his bike, looking down at me.

"You're out of shape!" he teased.

I didn't laugh.

With a bit more concern, he asked, "Are you ok?"

"I'm fine," I lied. "I just need a second to catch my breath."

He teased me again. "You aren't used to being pushed so hard. You've been slacking off all these years, riding with your girlfriends!"

His accusation stung, but I refused to take the bait. I pretended to shrug it off, turning the blame back onto him. "I'm fit enough, but this isn't a race. Mountain biking is supposed to be fun, not a hammer fest. I've had enough for today. Let's go back to the car and go home for lunch."

Facundo didn't argue. When we returned to the parking lot I felt better and had put the incident completely behind me. I pulled out my phone and snapped a photo of Facundo, wanting a memento of our first mountain-bike ride together. When I uploaded it to Facebook, I saw I had several missed calls, and my voicemail was full. Much to Facundo's annoyance, I had a habit of putting my phone on silent and then forgetting to turn it back on again.

While Facundo drove, I listened to my messages on speaker.

"Hello, Kristina, this is the Vancouver General Hospital calling. We received your Holter test results and need to discuss them with you today. We need you to check yourself into the emergency room as soon as you get this message."

The next one was from my sister, Jan. She didn't sound panicked, just a bit confused. "Hey, Kris. I got a call from the hospital. I guess you have me down as your next of kin? They say that they can't reach you. What is this all about?"

I turned to Facundo and tried to reason my way out of going to the hospital. "It can probably wait. I don't want to waste our whole day in the emergency room because of a misunderstanding." Facundo didn't say anything, so I pressed the point. "I've been living with this since August. I know how to recreate the symptoms, and I also know how to make them go away again. It isn't anything to worry about."

"Really?" he countered. "Then what was that all about on the ride today? Why did you have to stop and lie down if you aren't out of shape?" He knew I would prefer to blame my near-fainting spell on a problem beyond my control rather than being unfit to ride with him. "No, if they saw something on your test results and say that you should go in, then we're going in."

We drove the rest of the way in silence. When we arrived home, Facundo hosed down the muddy bikes while I bathed Naiya. We took our time showering and eating lunch before driving to the hospital.

***

We sat in the waiting room for five hours.

Periodically, I was summoned for blood tests and to offer more information, until we were the only two left sitting side by side in the orange plastic chairs. Finally, my name was called to see the doctor. When I stood up alone, they suggested that I may want to bring Facundo with me.

Instead of showing us to a bed with a curtain around it, an intern brought us into a private room and closed the door behind us.

He looked very young and earnest. I felt compelled to say something to help him relax, but I couldn't think of anything. I was tired and wanted to go home.

He asked me to sit down and then began to speak slowly. "The 24-hour Holter test showed a dangerous arrhythmia. This is why we asked you to come in today. You know those feelings you have when you feel faint? Well, that's your heart going into ventricular tachycardia. Also, your blood test confirmed that you have very high levels of troponin, an enzyme released after a heart attack or myocardial injury."

I flinched and told him about having to lie down in the dirt that morning during our mountain-bike ride. "Was that ventricular tachycardia?"

"It is possible. Troponin can remain in the bloodstream for up to two weeks, so I can't say for sure. But, Kristina, this is an extremely dangerous arrhythmia. There is a high probability that if this happens again, your heart may stop and won't start again. You are fortunate that it hasn't happened yet."

The intern paused for a moment and allowed this information to sink in.

Then he continued, "We can't let you leave today. We are going to admit you for observation over the weekend."

I no longer felt sorry for him and didn't hesitate when I told him no. "I have to be exercising at my maximum intensity to replicate those symptoms. If I stay here, you won't see anything. It will be a complete waste of time. Plus, haven't all the specialists gone home for the long weekend? No. I'm not staying."

He looked surprised. I don't think he expected me to argue. But he pulled himself together and attempted to assert a higher authority. "The cardiologist on call has informed me that we have to admit you."

I stood up from the chair and, attempting to appear confident, demanded, "I want to speak to the cardiologist."

The nurse escorted us back into the waiting room to wait for the cardiologist. Facundo wasn't as confident about my decision.

"Kristina, these doctors have spent years studying medicine. Maybe we should listen to them if they think that you need to stay."

The nurse nodded her approval. I wavered for the briefest moment, considering Facundo's logic. I understood that if someone with more education and knowledge told you to do something, you should listen. But Facundo wasn't the one being forced to stay, and he didn't know what I was feeling.

Again, I repeated myself, "But … I don't feel anything when I'm not exercising. Lying in a hospital bed is a waste of time."

Overhearing this, the nurse chimed in. "Exercising? Oh, I stopped that years ago. I used to train in the gym every day and finally realized that exercise was a waste of time. I feel so much better now."

I looked at her in disbelief. At first, I thought she was joking, but she wasn't laughing. There was so much I wanted to say to this, but now wasn't the time. Instead, I chose to ignore her and focus on my current situation.

"No," I said again. And feeling like a parrot, I repeated what I'd been saying since our drive home from mountain biking. "I've been living with this for months; a few more days isn't going to make any difference. I'm not staying."

I never did see the cardiologist on call that day. After much discussion, I signed an AMA (Against Medical Advice) form, relieving the hospital of any responsibility if anything went wrong. I was permitted to go home but promised to follow up with the cardiologist the following week.

CHAPTER 6

PLUMBERS AND ELECTRICIANS

That Thursday, October 15th, 2015, Facundo and I left the cardiologist's office in a daze. It was just too surreal to believe. We had heard the doctor's words and understood their meaning but could not accept that they were meant for me.

The cardiologist informed us that my heart had an electrical problem; precisely what it was, he didn't know. The diagnosis was beyond his specialty. He was a plumber, and what I needed was an electrician, was what he said. He sent me for an MRI and referred me to the BC Inherited Arrhythmia Program (BCIAP) at St. Paul's Hospital for further testing.

But whatever the problem was, I was screwed. Those were not the cardiologist's words exactly. Still, according to "the plumber," my only three treatment options for any electrical problem were medication, an implantable cardioverter defibrillator (ICD), or a heart transplant. The cardiologist educated me on the probability of success of each option as they pertained to me personally.

"With a resting heart rate of under 50 beats per minute and low blood pressure, you wouldn't tolerate the appropriate medication's side effects. If you had an ICD inserted, your daily physical training and exercise would prematurely set it off. But you would make an excellent candidate for a heart transplant. I can only imagine how excited the surgeons would be to perform a heart transplant on you. It's a rare opportunity to operate on someone so healthy."

I looked at him in complete incredulity. Not only were his words too much to absorb, but I was shocked at how much pleasure he took in delivering them. He didn't even have the decency to talk in that soft gentle voice that newscasters use when announcing horrible events. All I could think was, *This has to be a mistake. I need to find a new cardiologist.*

A few days after the meeting, I got a call that my MRI was scheduled for October 30th, just two weeks away. How had my problem become so urgent that I could get an appointment that quickly? The Canadian medical system prioritizes the most urgent cases, ensuring those people get the necessary care first. I didn't feel my case was bad enough to meet this criteria, but I didn't argue.

For the next two weeks, I was sent for numerous tests: several echocardiograms, multiple ECGs, and blood work. Whenever a nurse read my chart, they often exclaimed, "Wow, ventricular tachycardia; I have only ever seen that in the emergency room before we put on the paddles!"

I wasn't sure how I was supposed to take this bit of information. Should I be excited that I was still alive or scared I could die suddenly? I felt neither and decided not to respond.

A few days after the MRI, I received a phone call from Dr. Bregman. I had been walking Naiya along Kits Beach, enjoying the cool weather. When I heard my family doctor's voice, I felt alarmed. After a brief introduction, he launched into the reason for the call. The MRI and test results did not look good, and I needed to prepare myself for an ICD.

As I listened to his concerns, I thought back to "the plumber" and his warning that an ICD in someone as active as me would prematurely set the device off. I had no intention of living in fear of being shocked every time I went for a bike ride. But I also didn't want to have an argument with my family doctor about it. I really liked Dr. Bregman. He was kind, empathetic, and thorough. I also knew he worried about his patients, and I didn't want him to worry about me. Ever since I had dropped off the 24-hour Holter monitor, everyone was afraid that I would drop dead the next time I rode my bike or did any form of exercise. Reminding them that I had been living with this condition, whatever it was, for at least seven months didn't offer them any reassurance.

Either way, I was confident that the specialists at the BCIAP would figure it out and an ICD wouldn't be necessary. My appointment was only two weeks away, so to appease Dr. Bregman, I promised him I wouldn't exercise hard until then.

CHAPTER 7

ANIMAL IN A ZOO

On November 18th, 2015, the hour before my appointment with the electrophysiologist (EP) at the BCIAP, I was scheduled for a stress test. When I arrived, I asked the technician if I could do the test on the exercise bike instead of the treadmill. I explained that I had stopped running competitively a few years ago and there was no way I could force my heart rate high enough to reproduce the same symptoms as I could on a bike. The technician rolled her eyes at my arrogance and answered flatly, "If the doctor ordered a stress test on the treadmill, that's what we're doing."

So, with my breasts flopping under the hospital gown, I ran as hard as possible until she told me she had seen enough and I was done. As I had predicted, nothing happened.

After the stress test, Facundo and I waited for the results in the BCIAP examining room. Knowing that the arrhythmia was the only thing the doctors wanted to see, it felt like we were wasting precious time. I was frustrated that it hadn't worked, especially since I knew exactly how to replicate the symptoms. Facundo attempted to calm me by reminding me everyone was on my side, doing their best to find a solution for me. It made no sense to let out my frustration on the medical team, who were the very ones trying to help me.

His reprimand was cut short when the door opened and four doctors filed in: an electrophysiologist named Dr. Laksman, a cardiologist fellow named Dr. Morris (not his real name), a genetic counsellor, and one other person. I wasn't sure of her specialty. I should have felt relief knowing that I had so many people helping me, but with five pairs of eyes trained on me, I felt like I was suffocating.

As they delivered the news I had been dreading, I did my best to slow my breathing and calm my irritation. The treadmill test and the 24-hour Holter monitor hadn't provided enough information. They needed to witness the ventricular tachycardia (VT) for themselves. They couldn't give me a diagnosis or treatment plan until I did more tests and, yes, I would have to repeat the stress test.

Attempting not to sound arrogant — I was the patient after all — I told them that I could only replicate the VT on a bike. During my treadmill test, I remembered watching a frail man riding the ancient bike on the other side of the lab. He had barely been moving the pedals, but his face had been contorted in pain, and he'd been sweating with the effort. The bike wasn't designed for an experienced cyclist. After years of abuse, it was in worse condition than those at the local community centre. I knew that attempting the typical stress test on the lab bike would have its own complications and ultimately fail as well. In addition, the lab technician would never allow me to ride the bike long enough to reproduce the symptoms. I told them all this and offered to bring in one of my own bikes and a trainer, but they insisted that we use their lab bike. At this point, any guise of patience was gone. Ignoring Facundo, who was shooting me daggers with his eyes, I continued to argue with the team.

"Fine. I'll do the stress test on the lab bike, but if you want me to replicate the symptoms, we have to do it my way," I said.

To my surprise, with Dr. Morris' supervision, they agreed.

***

Exactly one month later, we were back at St Paul's Hospital for the second stress test. This time I was familiar with the drill. I went into the changing room, removed my clothing from the waist up, slid my arms into the sleeves of an oversized hospital gown, and tied it up in the front. Returning to the lab, I sat on an examining table and watched the lab technician place the sticky pads onto my bare chest. Once he was finished, I bunched up the long gown and tied it into a tight knot at my waist so it wouldn't become tangled between my legs and the bike.

Setting up the bike took a bit of time. I adjusted the seat height to fit my leg length and moved the handlebars as low and forward as possible. I climbed on and off the bike several times, readjusting everything by the tiniest measurements until I was satisfied. When I had determined that nothing could possibly hamper my performance, I climbed on and placed my feet on the pedals. Bending down, I tightened the toe straps, locking my running shoes into place.

I had known my audience would have a limited attention span, for which I had come prepared. Before arriving at the hospital, I rode on my bike trainer for thirty minutes, warming up the same way I had done for the FTP test less than two months prior.

Along with Dr. Morris were two lab technicians and four or five medical students. The room was packed with white coats trying to look at me and the rickety old exercise bike. I felt like an animal in a zoo.

"Since we have so many people, can my boyfriend come in?" I asked. "He will motivate me, help me reproduce the symptoms faster."

"No, he may get in the way if…" Dr. Morris didn't finish his sentence. *If anything happens.* The words hung between us, unspoken.

Since I was already testing their patience by requesting a unique testing procedure, I didn't push it further. I would have to do this alone. I could do that.

I turned to the technician and, trying my best not to sound bossy, I gave him my instructions. "Start the test at 200 watts, please."

Then I turned my attention back to the bike. I took in a long, deep, slow breath, mentally preparing myself for the pain that I was about to put myself through.

The lab bike's computer had a timer, calories, and cadence. I focused on the cadence, which calculates how fast the pedals turn, measured as revolutions per minute (rpm). My goal was to hold 95 rpm until I felt like I would pass out, which I now knew would replicate the VT they were looking for.

The technician confirmed that the machine was set to 200 watts, but the tension felt much easier than that. I watched my cadence climb well past 110 rpm. Not wanting to exhaust my legs before I could show them the VT, I silently reprimanded myself, took in another deep breath, and slowed my legs down to 95 rpm.

Once my cadence was under control, I asked the technician to, "Bring it up."

Immediately, the tension under my pedals increased. Now I had something to push against. I ignored all the people hovering around me and focused on the cadence. Silently, I kept repeating the mantra, *Hold it steady, Kristina. Hold it steady.*

The only sound was the wind going through the bike's front wheel and my heavy breathing. I watched the timer as the minutes continued to add up. Without taking my eyes off the display, I could sense that the students were becoming bored, shifting on their feet. Watching someone ride a bike only becomes interesting when they win or crash. I had to deliver the show they had come for.

"Bump it up!" I demanded again. "I need more tension."

Again the technician obliged.

Either the bike was slow to respond, or he bumped it up too quickly, but suddenly I went from riding at a cadence of 95 rpm down to 5 rpm. I could barely move the pedals, but still, I tried. The students started to pack up their clipboards and walk out of the room.

Dr. Morris, who had never left my side, told me the test was over. "You're done, Kristina."

He tried to help me off the bike, but I had a vice-like grip on the handlebars, and with my feet strapped to the pedals, he couldn't budge me.

"NO!" I screamed. "I'm not done! It's the bike, not me. I can do more. I can do more. I'm not leaving until you see what I'm talking about."

The students turned around, retracing their steps back into the room. Now they had a show to watch. Dr. Morris had me by both shoulders and was attempting to drag me off the bike. I understood I was acting like a toddler who wasn't getting what she wanted, but I was beyond caring. I knew nothing more would happen with my treatment if I didn't show them the VT today. It had to be today.

"Just give me five more minutes!" I pleaded.

Dr. Morris let go of my shoulders and agreed. "You have five more minutes, but that's it. Then you're done."

Through the open door of the lab, I could see Facundo standing on his tiptoes, trying to look over the students' heads to see why I was screaming. But he didn't barge his way in as I had hoped. He remained stationed just outside the door, as he'd been instructed.

I was annoyed with Facundo for not insisting on coming into the room — for not helping me. In my mind, I imagined he had ignored the doctors and had pushed his way to my side. I pictured him standing beside me, yelling at me to ride harder. Remembering his frustration when I couldn't replicate the symptoms at home, I thought, *I will show him. I will show all of them.*

"Bring it back down to 225 watts," I barked.

Then, like I had reproduced the symptoms with the 24-hour Holter monitor test, I ignored the display, put my head down, and pounded on the pedals. I was furious that they were giving up on me so soon and resented that I had to repeat a test I had already done.

Within two minutes, the anger, heat, and exertion all combined into the perfect recipe for the VT they were looking for. When the machines started beeping furiously, setting off alarms everywhere, I sat up and smiled in triumph. I had done it.

Nobody in the room applauded my effort. With quick efficiency, everyone moved into position. Within seconds, I was off the bike and laid down on a bed. I wondered how they removed the toe straps so quickly. I looked around in amusement as everyone wore looks of panic. I told them my racing heart was nothing to worry about; it would pass in a moment. I had done this a dozen times on the bike, and it always passed. But they weren't listening to me anymore. I seemed to be the only one who was happy with my achievement. I stopped protesting and let them run around doing what they needed to do. Closing my eyes, I coaxed my body back into a relaxed state, slowing my heart rate with each controlled breath.

When my heart rhythm stabilized, the students left, and Facundo was allowed in. He was the only one who congratulated me for showing them the VT they wanted to see. Facundo knew me.

When I had dressed again, Dr. Morris took us into a private room and closed the door.

"Kristina, you have an arrhythmia coming from the right ventricle. Dr. Laksman would like to do a procedure called a cardiac ablation. In this procedure, he will attempt to destroy the cells causing your abnormal rhythms. We have seen some good results with this procedure and think you may be a good candidate. But," he warned us, "as you've proven today, an immense amount of adrenaline and the perfect conditions are required to reproduce the arrhythmia. If they can't locate the problem areas in the procedure, they won't be able to do anything. In addition, even if they locate the problem areas, there is no guarantee that the ablation will solve all your problems. We don't want you to get your hopes up, but we think it's worth a shot."

Despite Dr. Morris' warnings, my hopes were indeed high. If there was even the slightest chance they could fix my heart and I could return to riding in the spring, I was up for it. I didn't need any time to think about it and agreed to the procedure immediately.

CHAPTER 8

DIAGNOSIS DENIAL

Navigating the medical system was confusing. In a few short months, I had met with so many specialists that it was unclear who was in charge of my care. Or was it up to me? The first cardiologist, who had read my initial 24-hour Holter monitor, suggested I would need someone to "oversee my file so I wouldn't get lost in the system." If that was true, I wanted to find a cardiologist who was experienced in treating athletes and was less excited about the prospect of a heart transplant.

I started shopping for a cardiologist who could oversee my care. One week before my ablation surgery, I booked an appointment with a sports cardiologist. My hope was that the ablation procedure would fix the arrhythmia and the sports cardiologist would provide a training plan so I could resume exercising.

I went into the meeting feeling positive. I was sure that the sports cardiologist would find a way to get me back to training. So when he announced, "Obviously, you have ARVC," I sat dumbfounded. If he had just said, "Kristina, you have ARVC," I might have believed him. But the "obviously" part caught me off guard and confused me. If the diagnosis was so obvious, why was this the first time I was hearing of it? And from a specialist who I had met just 20 minutes ago? Why hadn't Dr. Bregman, Dr. Laksman, or anyone at the BCIAP informed me of this diagnosis? Did everyone else already know and forget to tell me? Or had the entire diagnosis gone over my head during one of the many doctors' appointments when I felt so frustrated I stopped listening? How was it possible to miss your own diagnosis?

I looked down at my hands. I could feel tears threatening to spill over and I didn't want the sports cardiologist to see me cry. It took all my mental strength to make it through any conversation concerning my heart without crying. When I gained enough self-control, I looked back up and stared at the doctor, wondering how he could be so blunt. He was an athlete — both a runner and a cyclist. He should have known how devastating a diagnosis like this was for an athlete. Did doctors become so numb to their work that they forgot their patients were human? Or was I being a difficult patient and not listening?

I knew what ARVC was. The week prior, I had shown my MRI report to my friend, Dr. Ali Zentner. The report had stated "no signs of ARVC," which Ali had told me was a good thing and a relief. Even so, I had googled the acronym. What harm was there in researching a disease I didn't have?

Facundo had been working on his computer when I suddenly burst into tears. He thought that something was wrong with my heart. I shook my head, no, and turned the screen towards him so he could read the definition himself. According to several different websites, I learned that arrhythmogenic right ventricular cardiomyopathy (ARVC) is an inherited progressive heart condition in which the muscle of the heart's right ventricle is replaced by fat and/or scar tissue. This breakdown of communication increases the risk of an abnormal heartbeat (arrhythmia) and sudden death. I clicked on a few other websites.

"It says that in some cases, the patient will require a heart transplant!" I sobbed.

Facundo had wrapped me in his arms and reassured me that I was looking at the worst-case scenario. "That isn't going to happen to you. You don't have a rare genetic disease, and you aren't going to need a heart transplant."

But Facundo had been wrong. And now this one sentence, "Obviously, you have ARVC," destroyed any hopes I had of finding a cure. I stammered that I couldn't possibly have ARVC. Exercise was my life, my passion, and my entire identity. I was a cycling coach. I couldn't do my job without exercising.

The room suddenly felt stifling, and I could feel my face burning red-hot. I removed my sweater, hoping the cardiologist would see my shoulder muscles and rethink his initial prognosis. *Oh, I didn't realize she was such an athlete. Ok, we can give her a different exercise prescription.*

Wasn't that what he was supposed to do? Help athletes with their heart problems? But he didn't care about my muscles or what I would have to give up. Ignoring my angry glare, the doctor walked me through study after study, explaining why I needed to stop all exercise immediately and FOREVER. The only two acceptable sports were lawn bowling and golf.

Listening to the case studies only irritated me more. With each one I launched a new argument, attempting to prove that I was a unique case and those studies didn't apply to me. I had booked the appointment hoping he would provide a training plan, not tell me to stop exercising. Although I assumed he had read my chart, I summarized all the medical appointments and tests I had undergone in the last four months. It was a weak attempt to prove that he, the sports cardiologist, was wrong.

My MRI results reported no signs of ARVC. My DNA blood tests were inconclusive for the disease. None of my family members had the disease, nor did they have any gene markers for it. But none of this information seemed relevant enough for the doctor to second-guess his diagnosis. Again, he was a plumber. I needed an electrician.

The sports cardiologist was done trying to convince me. "There is nothing more I can do to help you," he said, ending the appointment.

I felt hopeless. The Kits Energy outdoor bike workouts would start up again in exactly one month. I had run out of time and would not be in any shape to ride or coach this season. I thought of Dr. Laksman, the electrophysiologist at the BCIAP. He was my last and only hope of finding a cure and possibly getting me back on my bike again. The moment

I left the hospital, I phoned the BCIAP clinic, requesting to speak directly to Dr. Laksman.

One hour later, he actually returned my call. I was driving Naiya to the woods, but when I saw the caller ID, I pulled the car over to answer. I was so upset that I was shaking. Without any preamble, I demanded, "Why would the sports cardiologist say that I have ARVC when you haven't said anything like that to me?"

Dr. Laksman's voice was calm on the other end of the line, as he answered slowly. "Kristina, we can't be 100 percent certain, but on a scale of black and white, you're very dark grey. You have many of the symptoms and characteristics of the disease — it's the most probable conclusion."

He paused for a moment as I sobbed on the other end of the line, then began again. "We don't really know if exercise will make your specific condition worse, but past studies have shown that it will."

This was my worst nightmare. In every dangerous sport I had engaged in, just before I jumped off a rock or pulled off some crazy stunt, the last thought that calmed my nerves and convinced me to make the leap was: *Hopefully, I die quickly.* I know that sounds insane, immature, and ignorant. Still, my rationale was that if I was dead, I wouldn't know it and would already be enjoying the afterlife, whatever that was.

But this time I hadn't jumped or done anything crazy. I had lived the last 40 years trying to be healthy. My plan was to continue racing and working into my 80s, maybe even 90s. *I'm a personal trainer, dammit. Shouldn't I know how to care for my own body?*

I needed Dr. Laksman to spell it out for me.

I asked, "How serious is this?"

"Kristina, I don't usually do personal phone calls, but I'm calling you, aren't I? That means it's serious," he said.

I wished he wouldn't beat around the bush and instead tell me directly. I continued questioning him.

"Why didn't you tell me?"

He took a deep breath and said, "Even if your problem has a different name, we would still treat you the same. This doesn't change anything."

It doesn't change anything? I thought. *It changes everything!*

"Kristina, why don't we see what happens after the ablation next week?" he said. "Then we can discuss other treatment options."

I hung up and continued crying until Naiya began licking my tears.

Later, as we walked in the woods, I watched Naiya chase squirrels in and out of the trees. She was turning seven that year but showed no signs of slowing down. I thought of all the weekends we had spent mountain biking, snowshoeing, hiking, cross-country skiing, and trail running. We would play for hours before either of us got tired. If the plumbers were correct, we would never do any of that again. I wandered aimlessly through the trails, feeling completely alone.

By the time we had finished the walk and returned home, I had descended into full-blown depression and was intent on taking everyone I loved down with me. I walked into the apartment and went straight for the office, starting my tears all over again. Facundo was at his desk, and when he saw me he immediately wrapped me in his arms while I sobbed out the story of my appointment with the sports cardiologist and his diagnosis.

After listening to the whole story, Facundo pulled away. Forcing my chin up to look at him, he said, "Kristina, we'll manage our way through this together. We'll figure it out. But … but I'm not going to tolerate you feeling sorry for yourself all the time. I understand this is awful, and you don't deserve it, but life isn't fair."

Facundo's words stung. Why wasn't he comforting me when it was apparent I needed his support? Leaning back into him, I buried my head in his shoulder. I needed time to sift through his words and my emotions. I felt that I had a right to feel sorry for myself and I didn't want to feel brave. But the more I thought about it, the more I realized he was right. The diagnosis was a lousy card to be dealt, but it wouldn't go away. I wasn't sure how we would deal with it, but I knew I didn't want to do it alone.

I also knew that at that moment, I was standing with my toes peeking over the edge of a bottomless pit of self-pity, depression, and resentment. If I permitted myself to slide just a little way down that embankment, there would be no stopping it. I would destroy everything I had built and loved, including my relationship with Facundo.

CHAPTER 9

LIVING IN A BETA-BLOCKER FOG

The morning after my appointment with the sports cardiologist and my "obvious" diagnosis, Facundo's alarm went off at 6:15 a.m. It was Saturday, but he was working the day shift at the firehall. The moment Facundo rolled out of bed and put his feet on the floor, Naiya jumped in, taking his place. She curled her body into a tight ball, landing with her spine directly in contact with mine, and we both went back to sleep.

After the stress test on the bike, Dr. Laksman had prescribed a low dose of bisoprolol to prevent future arrhythmias. Bisoprolol is a beta-blocker which lowers blood pressure and blocks the action of epinephrine on the heart. The first cardiologist had warned me that I would not tolerate this medication well. He was correct.

The side effects were brutal. Previously, my resting heart rate averaged 50 bpm, which is already low, but with the beta-blockers it hovered in the mid-30s. With my blood moving at a snail's pace through my arteries, I could never stay warm. While working in the air-conditioned gym, I wore two layers of tights, a big puffy vest, and a toque, and still my clients commented that my hands and lips were frequently blue. My blood pressure was so low that I felt lightheaded most of the time and had a constant headache, which morphed into a migraine when I was overly tired or stressed. My brain felt foggy, making it difficult to concentrate. When I did attempt to exercise, the medication wouldn't allow me to raise my heart rate over 100 bpm. Anytime I got close, I felt dizzy, nauseous, and gasped for air. Dr. Laksman said my body would eventually adjust, but I wondered what I would do if it didn't. There was no way I could continue living like this.

When I awoke again, I glanced over at the clock. It was already 8 a.m. I never slept in on weekends and I felt guilty. Before my diagnosis, by 8 a.m. I would already have walked Naiya, eaten breakfast, and would be preparing for a long ride with friends. For as long as I could remember, I always had a surplus of energy — until now. The beta-blockers had sucked every bit of motivation and energy out of me.

What do people do with their weekends if they don't exercise? What do people do for fun? I wondered. I wanted to stay in bed all day, but Naiya needed to go out. I dragged myself up, made coffee, and looked at the selection of breakfast options. Nothing seemed appealing. The beta-blockers made me nauseous, and with so little exercise, I barely had an appetite anymore. I poured my coffee into a travel mug, pulled on an old pair of tights and a sweater, and left the house.

On our drive to Pacific Spirit Park, I passed several groups of cyclists heading out for their long Saturday-morning ride and felt stabs of jealousy. Every one of my friends and most of my clients would be riding that morning. I wanted to be riding as well, not walking my dog. Stepping out of the car, I watched wistfully as another large group of cyclists whizzed by me. A few riders recognized me and waved. They looked so happy. I waved back and attempted to smile. The familiar buzz of wheels all spinning at once felt like pure torture. I knew how good that feeling of riding in unison was. Swallowing back my tears, I turned my back to the riders and marched into the woods.

I power-walked as quickly as my heart would allow. The fast pace was partly out of habit and partly out of guilt for not being able to exercise like I felt I should be. *If I can't ride, the least I can do is walk.* I chose a route that I knew would take me two hours to complete, then put an earbud into one ear and started an episode of my favourite podcast, *The Moth*. Listening to someone else's problems helped distract me from my own.

Within the first hour, I ran into two girlfriends from the gym. I could see them laughing and joking as they jogged towards me. When they noticed me, they stopped laughing and slowed to a walk. I didn't want them to stop. I didn't want to talk to anyone.

But, of course, I smiled and attempted to sound cheerful. "What a beautiful morning for a run!"

They looked at me sadly. "I heard about your heart problem," one said.

"That's a bummer," the other said.

"Yeah, thanks," I answered.

I didn't want to risk saying anything more as I wouldn't be able to hold back the tears if I did.

The girls continued by offering advice. "I have a friend who had a heart problem. He got a pacemaker and now he races Ironman."

Great! I thought. *Just what I want to hear — someone else's success story when I can barely make my way through a walk.*

I knew she was trying to be encouraging, to give me hope, but I wanted to scream that just because their friend was fine didn't mean I was ok.

"That's nice for him," I said. Not wanting them to see me cry, I added, "You two should keep running before you get cold."

They agreed, said goodbye, and jogged away. As soon as the girls were out of sight, my smile collapsed. I let the tears fall unchecked. Self-pity the size of an elephant began to swell up in my chest, creating a dull ache. How amazing it is that the heart can feel physical pain in so many ways.

After talking to the girls, I was too distracted to listen to *The Moth*. I turned off the podcast and thought about what I would do with my life if the doctors were right and I couldn't exercise anymore. *If I can't be a personal trainer and a cycling coach, what other job can I do? Maybe I should go back to school*, I thought. *But for what?*

When in doubt, call a friend… I phoned Rose. During the weekdays, Rose Cifelli and Cheryl Shkurhan alternated as my regular walking buddies. Both women lived between my apartment and the woods, so I would pick up one of them and drop them off again on my way home. During our walks they listened patiently while I panted up any slight incline and cried about the possibility of losing my job, identity, health, and the boyfriend I had hoped to marry. But no matter how devastating anyone's situation was, I knew how tiresome it could get for the listener. I made my best effort not to monopolize the entire hour.

But my need to talk to someone won over my fear of exhausting my friendship and, against my better judgement, I phoned Rose. She picked up on the second ring. I never even asked why she was still at home on a Saturday and not out riding her bike. Instead I blurted out, "I can't be a personal trainer anymore."

She wasn't surprised by my outburst. It was a continuation of a conversation we had been having that week. But she didn't sigh or get annoyed; instead, she encouraged me to continue talking by asking, "Why not? Lots of coaches don't do the actual sport anymore."

"But how do they manage?"

"What do you mean, how?" she countered. "At one time, they were experts in their field, so aren't they the most qualified people to coach?"

"No, I know how they do it, but I don't know why they would want to," I clarified. "Every morning when I walk into the gym to train clients, I want to scream in frustration because I want to do what they're doing. Every time I write an article about how to stay motivated to train, convince a client that life isn't over because they can't run for four weeks because of a sprained ankle, or when I encourage clients to run faster, or bike harder, I want to scream, 'IT'S NOT FAIR!'

How can I be motivating others when I'm jealous that I can't be doing what they're doing? Does a coach feel those things? Does a gymnastics coach get upset when she can't walk a balance beam anymore?"

I was really worked up now. Rose didn't interrupt me. She continued to listen patiently until I had exhausted myself. When I finished ranting, she sympathized but didn't have an answer for me. We said our goodbyes and I hung up the phone. My mental anguish had taken precedence over all other senses, rendering me blind to the beauty and sounds of the forest surrounding me. I finished my walk on auto-pilot.

When I returned home, I attempted to write in my journal, hoping it might help me see things more clearly. Staring at a blank page, I remembered Facundo's words from the previous night. I could let my resentment ruin everything that I had worked so hard to create, including my business, friendships, and most importantly, my relationship with Facundo. Or I could trust that something good would come out of this situation and my life would improve because of it.

I need to stay positive and not let this disease destroy my life, I reminded myself. I had no clue how that was possible, but I had to figure it out, and soon.

CHAPTER 10

PLAN A

My ablation procedure was scheduled for March 14th, 2016, at 11 a.m. The night before the surgery, I slept well for the first time in months. I was excited, feeling hopeful that this procedure would fix the arrhythmia, and I could finally move on with my life.

In the morning, I awoke as usual. Per the doctor's orders, I skipped breakfast and used the extra time to walk Naiya longer than usual. I arrived at the gym full of nervous energy and cheerfully reminded my clients that I would be away the following week, but not to worry; Elaine was covering for me so they wouldn't miss any workouts.

I had hired Elaine Reid in 2014, around the time Facundo and I had started discussing the possibility of having children. I didn't have any hormonal urges to have children, but I didn't want to take that opportunity away from him, if that was what he wanted. As Facundo weighed the pros and cons of having a family, I gave him a deadline. He had until I turned 40 to make a decision. After that, I wasn't willing to risk getting pregnant. In the meantime, I made plans and set up my company so it could continue to run without me, should I need to go on maternity leave.

Once my fortieth birthday had come and gone, instead of a maternity leave, I relied on Elaine's help more and more so that I could spend numerous hours in medical appointments. With her covering for me, I knew that my clients were in good hands and I didn't need to worry. I don't know how I would have managed if we had children to care for as well.

After working that morning, I drove back home to pick up Facundo. He was committed to supporting me and insisted on being with me, staying with me until I went into surgery. I was grateful he was by my side, especially as my 11 a.m. appointment time came and went. Five and a half hours later, they finally squeezed me in as the last surgery of the day.

Before the procedure, the nurse had informed me that, although I wouldn't be asleep, I would have enough anesthesia that I wouldn't remember anything. However, during the procedure, I had moments of clarity. I was aware enough to know that they weren't able to reproduce the arrhythmia. Believing that I had power over my body, I blamed myself. Later, Dr. Laksman told me I had gotten so upset with the news that it wasn't working that I had put myself into VT. Only then could they try to ablate some of the rogue cells.

I was devastated. As they rolled the stretcher out of the operating room, everyone on the fifth floor could hear me as I wailed at the top of my lungs, "I failed! I failed! I failed!"

Facundo heard me long before I entered the room. Panicked, he asked the nurse, "What is she talking about? What happened?"

The nurse patted him on the arm and reassured him, "Don't worry about it, dear. It's only the drugs talking. She did fine."

But Facundo knew me better than that. We both expected that this surgery would fix my heart, and he knew how disappointed I would be when it didn't. We hadn't thought of a Plan B.

I felt utterly spent. Every muscle in my body ached like I had raced two marathons back to back. I was still groggy and crying when Dr. Laksman came to my bedside to provide a summary of how things had gone. I had difficulty focusing, but he confirmed what I had suspected. Essentially, they couldn't fix me, and I was no further ahead than before. Dr. Laksman reminded me of his previous warning that the surgery wasn't a guarantee. He attempted to absolve me of my guilt, but it didn't help. I was angry, disappointed, and utterly annoyed with my body for not being stronger. I lay motionless and allowed the tears to fall. I couldn't think of anything beyond the fact that my body had failed me. I didn't look at Facundo or ask him what he was thinking. I was too absorbed in my pain.

Dr. Laksman was still talking and I tried to refocus my attention. His thick eyebrows were bunched together in an expression of concern and empathy and his warm brown eyes moved slowly between Facundo and me, trying to include both of us in the conversation.

"Kristina, in my opinion, having an ICD inserted would be the wisest and safest choice for you at this time."

I frowned back at him. I had already made it very clear to everyone that there was no way I would have a metal device inserted in my chest. Not today, not next week, not ever. I was only 40. A defibrillator was for old people, not for young athletes like me. Although I didn't ask him, I was also afraid of what Facundo would think, seeing a hockey puck poking against my skin, looking as though it would pop out at any moment. And what about my clients? Wouldn't they conclude that I wasn't fit to train them anymore? But what terrified me the most was that if I allowed the doctors to insert an ICD, I would be admitting that I had a problem that I could not fix. And I wasn't a quitter. I wasn't ready to give up yet.

Dr. Laksman continued. "You have told me that you don't want an ICD, but would you consider an implanted loop recorder?"

This caught my attention.

He explained that a loop recorder was half the size of his pinky finger. It would be inserted just under the skin on the left side of the chest, making the procedure quick and only requiring local anesthesia. The loop recorder wouldn't help me if I had an arrhythmia or if my heart stopped — it was simply a recording device. But when I had an episode, it would send the information back to the nurses' station via Bluetooth. If the nurse saw anything concerning, I would get a call and we would follow up with whatever treatment was necessary. Also, with my consent, the information would be used as research and also help future patients in similar situations.

Dr. Laksman must have been tired after a full day in surgery, but he remained patient and asked again, "Would you agree to have a loop recorder inserted?"

I looked over at Facundo to gauge his reaction to the idea, but I couldn't read his facial expression.

"This is your decision," he said.

Obtaining more information and learning more about what was wrong with me was what I wanted most. Again, I hoped that it would help me find a solution. I also reasoned that the device was small and nobody would see it. So, after a few moments of consideration, I turned back to Dr. Laksman and nodded in agreement. He smiled and said he would book the appointment for the procedure in the next few weeks.

At 8 p.m. the surgery was closing and the day nurses and Dr. Laksman were free to return home, back to their own lives. I would also be permitted to leave the hospital that day, but only after demonstrating that I could walk a few steps independently. They wheeled me out of the recovery room and into a temporary, shared room where they brought a dinner plate in for the patient in the bed next to me. The smell emanating from the tray made my stomach revolt. Facundo grabbed the puke tray, but I had nothing left to vomit. Over 24 hours had gone by since I last ate or drank. I wanted to go home and sleep in my own bed.

Determined to leave, I had Facundo help me to a sitting position. I sat on the edge of the bed and waited for the dizziness to settle. When the nurse made his next round, I managed to gain enough control of my limbs to stand and stumble forward. I took only a few steps, but it was enough. Satisfied, the nurse left, and Facundo grabbed me before I collapsed. He helped me dress and wheeled me down the hall, into the elevator, and through the hospital to the ER exit.

As he went to retrieve the car, he left me sitting in the wheelchair parked just inside the exit doors. Every few minutes the automatic doors would slide open with a loud whoosh. With each rush of cold air, I looked up to see who had arrived: a woman high on drugs, a man in a hospital gown stubbing out the last of his cigarette. Another whoosh, and this time I watched a man slowly wander inside, mumbling to himself. He did not belong in the hospital, but no one was around to stop him.

The man looked like he was homeless. As I judged him, I realized that I must look no better. My hair was a sweaty, knotted mess on top of my head. I was wearing loose grey track pants and an old sweater. I stank horribly.

Through half-closed lids, I continued to monitor the man. He made me nervous and I silently prayed that he would not take any interest in me. Swearing to himself, he continued to wander around the room. As he moved closer to me, my pulse quickened, and with it came a heavy, dull ache in the centre of my chest. I realized that I had no way to defend myself against this man or anyone who came through those doors. If I had to run, I was sure my heart would explode. I hated my weakness, vulnerability, and my dependence on Facundo.

I sank lower in the chair and tried to make myself invisible.

CHAPTER 11

IS IT WORTH THE RISK?

On April 29th, 2016, I had the loop recorder implanted. As Dr. Laksman had promised, the procedure was fast, simple, and painless. During the procedure Facundo waited on the other side of the privacy curtain. When it was done, the device was so small that it was barely visible. Within two days, the four neat stitches were already healing quickly and hidden under my tank top.

Since my diagnosis, it felt like my symptoms had gotten worse, which didn't make sense to me. Initially, I had to push myself to extremes to feel the symptoms and now they were happening almost any time I exercised. Facundo and I thought that maybe I had turned into a hypochondriac. Was it possible that I was creating the symptoms in my head? I decided to use the loop recorder to test this theory.

I went to my closet and searched through a dozen or so matching jerseys and shorts to find the ones I was looking for: a generic black and white cycling kit that didn't have my business name printed all over it. I didn't want anyone to recognize me.

I chose long black socks to match, and then gathered all the other items: helmet, gloves, sunglasses, a jacket in case of rain, and a fully charged Garmin. I tightened my cycling shoes, as I had done hundreds and hundreds of times since I was sixteen years old, and remembered a question that my aunt had asked me way back then.

"Do you really need all that stuff just to go for a bike ride?"

I knew her question was only meant to annoy me, and that she wouldn't understand if I attempted to explain, so I had ignored her. But in my head, I had screamed, "Absolutely, I need all this stuff! Without it, I'm just someone riding a bike. Only a true rider would understand the difference."

Growing up, nobody in my family or any of my friends understood why I ran, cycled, and swam for hours on end; why I would choose to wake up at 5 a.m. to do these things; or why I would prefer to ride my bike instead of driving a car. They all told me repeatedly, "You need to relax more."

But the teasing and words of warning only fuelled me to train harder and longer. The discipline of training gave purpose to my life and helped me build self-confidence. Ironically, although I was working hard, it was during exercise that I felt the most relaxed. To them exercise meant hard work, but for me exercising was fun. So yes, I needed all of this gear to go for an easy ride and test my loop recorder.

The day I chose was a beautiful spring afternoon with only a slight, cool breeze. I pumped up my tires and carried my white Cervelo R3 down the stairs and out of my apartment. Coasting the two blocks down to Kits Beach, I took in a deep, full breath of the wet, salty air and immediately felt at peace. Spring arrives early in Vancouver and already I could see people filling up the tennis courts; sweaty young men pushing and shoving on the basketball court; and the beach packed with tanned, barely clothed bodies jumping up to the volleyball net.

Riding parallel to the beach, I passed groups of runners, dog walkers, and the famous Kits Beach pool, not yet open for the season. I passed several other cyclists and thought, *All of these people on the courts, on the beach, on their bikes don't know me, but they would understand me. They would never ask me whether I needed all this stuff to go for a ride.*

When I arrived at Rose and Benny's house, they were already outside pumping up their tires, getting ready to go. We had planned a short 60-kilometre ride to Iona Beach, which isn't much of a beach but is famous for the 4-kilometre jetty stretching into the Strait of Georgia, and the pebbled beach where you can walk your dog undisturbed. The route is relatively flat, has very few turns, and hardly any traffic lights, making it a popular cycling route.

I met Benny Cifelli in the spring of 2007 when we were both members of the Leading Edge Triathlon Club. Benny is an animated Italian who not only talks with his hands — his whole body vibrates with his enthusiasm. He took his fitness seriously but not so seriously as to decline a beer after a workout.

I met Rose in January of 2009, during my first season volunteering for the Team in Training Society, a charity that raised money for leukemia and lymphoma research. I had been recruited to teach/coach about 50 novice participants — who had never participated in a triathlon before — to finish an Olympic-distance race. Some participants could barely swim, and others hadn't been on a bike since elementary school. From February to April, the coldest and wettest months in Vancouver, my job was to make sure each of them could swim 750 metres, bike 40 kilometres, and run 10 kilometres before the race cutoff time. In exchange for my time, I was provided a three-day trip to Hawaii where I would coach the participants during the event. I would love to say that my volunteer work was purely altruistic, but in truth, my primary goal was to gain experience as a triathlon coach and continue building my coaching business.

I met Rose on the first day of training. She was quiet, like she wished her five-foot-three frame was even shorter so nobody would notice her. I only knew that Rose was a two-time Ironman Canada athlete because her friend bragged about her achievements during our introduction. It was evident that Rose didn't need my coaching and I was nervous that she might criticize my methods. But Rose was slow to advise and gentle when she did. Observing how difficult it was for one person to manage so many people at various levels and abilities, Rose offered to help. I gave her the title of assistant coach, which offered no benefits, just a lot of work. She never asked for anything in return and for three years she helped me coach every workout. During that first season,

Rose also became my Ironman training buddy, and we soon became close friends.

With me being the shared link, Rose and Benny finally met each other. In June of 2010, the three of us travelled to France for a week-long cycling trip. Our apartment was at the base of Alpe d'Huez, and every day we left early in the morning, climbing two to three "cols" (mountain passes) in a day. It shouldn't have been a surprise when Rose and Benny soon started dating, and on February 12th, 2014, I had the privilege of standing as Rose's maid of honour at their wedding.

We laughed and joked, but we knew that today's ride was not a casual training ride. Benny was a few years shy of 60 and had suffered a mild stroke that fall. Since then, he hadn't been riding much, if at all.

As we pulled away from their house, Rose remarked, "I remember when we first met, I was faster than you, but that only lasted one season. Since France, it's been years since you last agreed to ride with us. If it wasn't for your heart problem, you wouldn't be riding with us slow guys today."

I ignored the jab because I knew she was right. After training for Ironman, I had turned into a bike snob. Unless I was coaching or working with a client, I only trained with cyclists who rode at a similar pace or who were faster than me. I should have taken the opportunity to apologize. Instead, I said nothing and just laughed, pretending it was a joke. I had abandoned my best friend and had let go of so many friendships just because they weren't fast enough to keep up. Now it was Rose who was waiting for me.

For most people, our riding styles are a reflection of our personalities. Rose strictly monitored her training zones and never got tempted to go any faster than her plan permitted; her cadence always steady and consistent. Benny was also an experienced rider, but he was far from consistent. Benny rode as hard as he could until he ran out of energy and then suffered for the rest of the distance. Although he realized the fault in this strategy, he couldn't stop himself. Sprinting ahead, he would even foreshadow the inevitable. "I'm only good for the first hour, and then I'm going to hurt," he always said.

Unless I was coaching, I rode competitively, trying to match the speed of whoever I was riding with. If they were faster than me, I would hold on for dear life until I blew up and couldn't hold the pace anymore. If it was just me and Rose riding alone, I would have been content to ride at her pace, but I couldn't help myself when someone in the group sprinted ahead.

This was how the trouble started that day.

Within the first 3 kilometres, as the three of us crested the hill just past Spanish Banks, Benny took off. Without thinking, I stood up on my pedals and caught onto his wheel. Together we sprinted east along Southwest Marine Drive like it was a 10-kilometre time trial, never once looking back. Benny could hear me close to his back wheel and increased his speed, but I was determined not to let him drop me. Before the Arthur Laing Bridge, we pulled over and stopped in a parking lot to catch our breath. We were breathing heavily but laughing hysterically. The small chase had released endorphins, and it felt so good.

After several minutes, Rose gently slowed to a stop in front of us. We stopped laughing as soon as we saw the frown burrowing lines in her forehead.

"What is wrong with you two?" she yelled.

Rose never yells.

I looked down at the ground. Benny started to blubber out lame excuses and apologies. "We couldn't help it, sweetie. Oh, Rosie, honey, you know me. I like to go fast right out of the gate. But you are right. We should stay together."

I didn't say anything. I was ashamed at my inability to exert any self-control.

Sliding in behind Rose, we left the parking lot in single file, allowing her to set the pace. When riding in single file, the first cyclist blocks the wind, creating a draft for anyone riding behind, allowing them to ride at the same speed using much less energy. Rose never remained angry for long, but we didn't dare pass her again. I looked down at my Garmin and saw that we were only one-quarter into the ride. It hadn't occurred to me that 60 kilometres might be too far of a distance for a test ride. In the past, 60 kilometres was considered a short distance, something that we would whip off as a recovery ride in just over two hours.

We were now on the flat stretch heading out to Iona Beach. The airport was on our left, the ocean was in front, and the Fraser River was on our right. It is a given that there is always a headwind in this section; the only question is which way — going out or coming back. Today the headwind was going out, so I remained firmly behind Rose. I focused on her legs as they flexed and extended in a steady, unbroken push-and-pull movement. My own legs were beginning to cramp, and I could feel my ever-constant headache intensifying into a migraine. I tried to relax my upper body, willed my mind to go numb, and attempted to ignore the dull ache spreading throughout my chest. My heart, which used to feel light, powerful, and strong, now felt like lead, weighing me down.

I was accustomed to not conceding to pain. It is a learned skill and necessary if you want to be fast at any sport. When I was racing, I embraced pain, because once the pain arrived, I could gauge my effort. If the pain was still tolerable, I knew I could push more. If I judged that I had reached my pain threshold, I would be satisfied with whatever outcome or podium placing I received.

But something had shifted. The pain I was now experiencing didn't feel right. It was not the same muscle ache of hard work or the familiar burn of lactic acid build-up. Lately, doing anything that required physical effort just felt hard. I finally understood what people meant when they said they didn't like exercise. If this was how they felt riding a bike, I wouldn't want to do it either. I felt remorse that I hadn't understood this sooner in my life and particularly in my career as a personal trainer.

Looking ahead, past Rose's shoulder, I spotted an ambulance parked on the side of the road. The accident must have happened some time ago as there wasn't anyone around — no cars, no bikes, just the ambulance. As we rode closer, we could make out two paramedics standing in the ditch on the right side of the road.

Rose signalled that she was slowing down. We broke up our line so we could all get a better view. As cyclists, getting hit by a car was always a probability but something we tried not to think about. We understood the risks but crossed our fingers that it wouldn't happen to us.

Slowly we rolled by the scene. The paramedics weren't just waiting; they were standing guard. Between them, lying on the ground, was a motionless body covered by a black blanket. Poking out of the bottom of the blanket were a pair of men's black cycling shoes.

I felt sick to my stomach. The throbbing in my head increased in intensity and it felt like I was pedalling through sand.

"Oh, fuck," Benny said.

"I can't believe it!" I responded stupidly.

Not that I couldn't believe that someone could die, but not so suddenly, and not on the day I was testing my own limits.

Rose said nothing.

Although I hadn't seen him, my imagination gave the dead man a face — an identity, and a family he had left behind. When he got dressed that morning, pumped up his tires, and greeted his riding friends, he had no idea these would be his last few hours.

"That could very well have been me," I said.

In my head, I was also thinking it could have been Benny as well, but he was denying that his stroke was anything serious, so I didn't say it.

Rose snapped back, "Oh, stop it! Stop thinking like that."

She didn't want to think that anyone she loved could die this way, and she definitely didn't want it said aloud.

As we rode away from the scene, I asked, "Why are we out here risking our lives when Benny and I have been told to take it easy?"

Benny argued, "You could die just crossing the street. Just because there's a risk to something doesn't mean you should stop doing it. We're all going to die some time. Isn't it better to die doing something you love?"

That's exactly what I would have said a few months ago, but now I wasn't so sure. Before, the risk of me dying on the bike depended on someone running into me or me losing control. Both were possibilities but didn't seem very likely. Now I realized that I could die just because I chased someone up a hill. I was feeling so many conflicting emotions all at the same time.

Riding had always been my happy place. But did I love riding so much that I would risk dying for it? Was it really worth it?

I looked to my friends for confirmation and asked, "Benny, you and I have been given a second chance. Shouldn't we listen to the doctors and maybe do something different?"

Benny ignored my question and rode on ahead of us.

I stayed behind Rose, trying to save as much energy as possible. I wanted to be at home, safe in my bed, and not still on the road, exhausting myself. Any ambition I previously felt to push through the fatigue and pain had vanished. I felt such sadness for the cyclist who would not be riding home that day. I wondered who he had left behind. Who were the people who would have to go on living without him?

The mood had turned somber. Nobody was laughing or joking now. Rose continued to ride in front, looking back every so often to ensure that she hadn't dropped me. Halfway up one of the hills, I finally had to stop. My heart rate was spiking out of control, and no amount of mental work or controlled breathing would lower it. I felt nauseous and lightheaded. All these feelings had become familiar, almost predictable. When Rose looked back and saw me bent over the front of my handlebars, gasping for air, she rushed back towards me. I could see the worry in her eyes, but my only thought was, *At least now the loop recorder will tell me if this is real or just all in my head.*

Back at home, I immediately uploaded my loop recorder data to the remote device which sat on my bedside table and sent the transmission to the BCIAP nurses' station. I had been given instructions to notify them whenever I felt symptoms, so they could correlate them with what was happening to my heart. Within 30 minutes, I received a phone call confirming that my symptoms were real. She said a bunch of long words that I didn't understand; multiple runs of VT, isolated and bigeminal PVCs, and non-sustained runs of VT at 214–222. All I heard was "ventricular tachycardia" and I knew that wasn't good. She informed me that Dr. Laksman would follow up with me the following week. I thanked her, hung up the phone, and crawled into bed. I wondered, *If my heart rate hadn't returned to its normal rhythm, could that have been me lying on the side of the road with my white Sidas cycling shoes poking out of the bottom of a black blanket?*

This thought alone should have been enough to scare me into quitting sports altogether. But I was convinced that I would be the exception to the rules of this disease.

CHAPTER 12

BREAKING POINT

I could no longer deny the fact that my heart wasn't strong enough or stable enough to race, train, or even coach my outdoor cycling club that season. Fortuitously, the previous winter I had hired three new coaches. With Facundo coaching two groups for me, I had all five groups covered. So I decided that my role would be to help the new coaches gain confidence and, as their assistant, I could ride with a different group each week without having to exert myself. My plan was to ride as sweep, following the slowest rider, and offer extra coaching to those who needed it.

Although the coaches knew about my heart condition, I hadn't told the riders, and worked hard to hide the fact that I was struggling to keep up the pace. But with each week I grew weaker and was more of a liability than an asset to everyone. Every night I would return home completely spent. Facundo asked me why I continued to torture myself. Egotistically, I was afraid that the club would fall apart without me. I also couldn't accept the fact that I was no longer physically capable of doing something that used to come so naturally.

Facundo assured me that my club would be fine without me. I had hired and trained competent and knowledgeable cycling coaches who were more than capable of working without me, and might actually appreciate not having me micromanage them. I hated the idea of supervising from the sidelines and not participating in the workouts, but it was the right choice — at least until I found a solution for my heart. *It'll just be for one season,* I promised myself. *I'll be back to coaching next year.*

I stopped coaching, but I didn't stop cycling. After the latest episode, which had happened while riding to Iona with Rose and Benny, Dr. Laksman changed my prescription from bisoprolol to sotalol. But exchanging one beta-blocker for another didn't improve the side effects. The medication still wouldn't allow my heart rate to go above 100 bpm, so even while riding a stationary trainer inside, I barely broke a sweat. Desperately clinging to the last shreds of my identity as a cyclist, I felt that this was better than nothing. Even though every forum, research paper, and Google search of ARVC cautioned me against doing any form of endurance training, I could not give it up. I couldn't comprehend how completely abstaining from exercise was good for me either.

It is scientifically proven that you can train your heart to do more work at a lower heart rate by building a larger aerobic base. This type of adaptation requires long hours of training at a very low heart rate. So I reasoned that if I logged enough easy miles, eventually, I could get back to long-distance riding. Whenever I had the tiniest bit of extra energy, I forced myself to pedal for 30-minute intervals on the trainer. I wanted to prove to everyone, but mostly to myself, that I was an outlier, exempt from the usual medical protocols assigned to ARVC patients.

And this was the reason why I registered for a 100-kilometre ride called the Tour de Whatcom in Washington State. I chose this specific event because it was out of the province and less popular than other events among my clients and friends. In addition, there weren't any prizes to be won and, more importantly, no timing chips — nobody could look up my finishing time online afterwards. I didn't want anyone I knew to bear witness to me gulping for air like a fish out of water whenever my heart rate raced too high, or to see how much fitness I had lost.

Facundo thought it was a terrible idea. He didn't understand why I needed to pay for an event to test my ability to ride. I knew it didn't make logical sense, but completing this event felt like it would allow me to reclaim my identity as an athlete. I begged Facundo to do this with me — for me — and he agreed to support me. Rose and Benny wanted to join as well, and Rose offered to ride as my domestique, which meant she would do all the work for me by riding in front of me, while I got all the glory of riding fast without putting in much effort.

On July 24th, 2016, Facundo, Rose, Benny, and I stood in the second wave at the start line of the Tour de Whatcom. The second wave meant that we wouldn't get caught up with the riders wanting to race the event, but we were ahead of the slowest recreational riders. When the gun went off, Benny charged like a racehorse out of the gate. We didn't see him again until after the finish. Rose and I slipped in behind Facundo as he set a gentle but quick pace for us to follow. We rode in single file, wearing matching head-to-toe Kits Energy attire and all the gear that went with being a cyclist.

The course wasn't difficult, no big climbs, and there was barely a headwind that day. On each of the hills, Facundo slowed his pace so I could gently ascend without expending too much effort. For the first few kilometres I was enthusiastic about my progress. I was doing it! I was riding in an event again with my boyfriend and friends. But the euphoric feeling didn't last long. On the first long climb, my heart started to flutter uncomfortably and I was forced to slow down. I felt like I was barely moving, crawling up the hill.

I felt pressure from the riders behind me to speed up. I looked over my shoulder and was shocked to see a long train of cyclists trailing behind me. But for some reason, no matter how slow I rode, nobody passed me. I was confused. Why would so many riders be riding this slow? I hadn't anticipated that I would hold anyone up and cringed with embarrassment. *Why aren't they passing me?*

I got my answer when a short man with his jersey stretched tight across his ample belly pulled up beside me and declared, "I'm feeling really good today, but there is no way I would pass you!"

I followed his gaze to look ahead at Rose and Facundo; both were experienced coaches and extremely fit. I understood the confusion. The man thought that we knew something about the course that he didn't.

At this point, I was gasping for air, but there was no way I would admit that to him. Throughout years of teaching spin classes and coaching on a bike, I had learned how to speak between the gasps while making it look effortless. The key was to keep the sentences short and only speak each complete sentence during the exhale so the pause for inhalation wasn't noticeable and the words didn't sound robotic.

I smiled at him, took in a massive gulp of air, and tried to make my voice sound casual as I answered. "Oh, no, you should definitely pass us! We are just out for an easy ride today."

He looked me up and down, and I could hear the doubt in his voice when he said, "But your easy ride is probably my hard ride."

I took in another gulp of air and exhaled, "No! No, please go ahead. We are going to slow you down if you stay behind us."

He still didn't believe me but slowly tested my theory and began pulling ahead. Building confidence, he moved past Rose, then Facundo, and disappeared over the ridge.

In any race, as soon as the gun went off, my attention narrowed and I became 100-percent focused on my performance. It is what I cherished most about racing — the feeling that nothing else mattered except that moment. Time was only relevant when it provided useful information such as speed, total elapsed time relative to the goal, and when it was time to eat and drink. But on this day, I couldn't focus. The minutes seemed to drag on and my legs felt heavier with each forced pedal stroke. My chest throbbed. But every time

Facundo rode back to check on me, I smiled brightly and exclaimed, "It is so great to be on a bike again with you!"

It had been my idea to ride this event. I refused to admit I had been wrong. But Facundo knew me well and could see the signs that I was suffering. He shook his head at my stubbornness and then moved back to the front.

We were halfway through the ride, and I was trying hard to focus on a mantra so I could forget my chest pain, when we rounded a corner and time did stop. Directly in front of us, straddling both lanes, sat an old grey four-door car flat on its hood. Every window had been smashed in, and glass was everywhere. Anything loose in the car was strewn across the road, including its passengers. As we surveyed the scene, we realized that it must have happened just moments before we had arrived. We did a quick scan of the road looking for bikes and any cyclist who might have been hit. My mind immediately went to Benny. But by some miracle, not a single cyclist was in the accident. It was just the one car and the three people who had been thrown from it.

On the ground, a few feet from the vehicle, a middle-aged man lay on his side, unconscious. Beside him knelt a thin, small woman screaming hysterically for him to wake up. Slightly behind them was a teenage boy rocking himself back and forth silently.

As a firefighter, Facundo moved into autopilot. He attended to the unconscious man first. The man was breathing and had a pulse; someone called 911 and, while we waited for the ambulance, Facundo stayed beside him, monitoring his vitals. I worked to control traffic. Glass was strewn all over the road and I warned approaching cyclists to get off their bikes and carry them across the accident scene to protect their tires from punctures.

The scene felt chaotic. Every so often, the injured woman would go into complete hysterics. She repeatedly tried to shake the man to wake him up. Facundo had to physically restrain her so that she couldn't cause the man any further damage, which only caused her to scream louder. Every time she screamed, I could feel my own heart rate rising. I felt sick. I wished I hadn't registered for the event. Facundo had been right; it was a terrible idea. If we had been just a few minutes faster, the car could have crashed into one of us, or maybe all of us. With so many bikes on the road that day, it was a miracle that not a single cyclist had been hit.

If it wasn't for me, we wouldn't even be here. I couldn't believe that this was happening to me again. I thought back to the time I was testing my loop recorder with Rose and Benny and we had come across the cyclist lying on the side of the road at Iona, who I later found out died from a heart attack. Again I wondered if training and racing were worth dying for. What was I doing out here? Why was it so important for me to ride this event? I didn't know the answers to those questions anymore.

Finally, the ambulance arrived, and we were able to leave. I clipped into my pedal, but before pushing off I looked back at the three strangers one last time and wondered how their lives would unfold. Would the man live, or was this his day to die?

Rose and I resumed our positions behind Facundo, who was now setting a slightly faster pace to make up for the lost time. But my heart rate was still racing high with adrenaline and I couldn't keep up with them. I didn't want to continue riding, but quitting or taking a shortcut never entered my mind. Whenever I fell too far behind, Facundo circled back and rode directly in front of me to break the wind. Once I caught up to Rose again, he would return to the front and set the pace, just a little faster.

After the fourth, fifth, or maybe twentieth time that Facundo had circled back, he pulled up beside me and, looking annoyed, asked, "Can't you ride any faster?"

"Do you think I like this?" I shot back. "Do you really think that if I could ride any faster, I would choose to ride this slow?"

I was so angry that I was screaming. Rose pulled ahead to give us some privacy. As my anger mounted, my speed slowed even more. I couldn't ride and talk simultaneously, let alone scream. Without a word and with no effort, Facundo took off and left me alone on the hill. I wasn't angry at him. I was angry with myself. I was angry that this event had been a failure. I was angry because it was clear to me now that I was no longer a rider. I was now just someone who rode a bike, and I could barely do even that.

I struggled to keep the bike moving forward, but my heart couldn't keep up. Everything inside me was screaming for me to stop. My chest burned. My head was pounding. My legs felt like lead sticks that refused to move at my command. And now I was alone on the empty road.

Dr. Laksman's words echoed in my mind. *"Your heart could stop at any moment."* I wondered if this would be the day I died. I didn't really believe it, but does anyone really believe they will die, until they take their last breath? I started to panic, but this only made my heart beat faster, so I willed myself not to think about death or dying.

After I had the loop recorder inserted, Dr. Laksman had asked me to buy an external defibrillator. Even though I had successfully gotten myself out of dangerous arrhythmias in the past, he was doubtful that I would always be so lucky. He wanted me to carry it at all times, especially when exercising. But if I thought an ICD labelled me as helpless, I definitely wasn't willing to carry around an external defibrillator. Besides, if Dr. Laksman was correct and my heart did stop, I felt that it was unfair of me to ask Facundo or any of my friends to revive me. What if they weren't successful? They would blame themselves when, in fact, it would be my fault for not getting the ICD. I did not want to place that responsibility on anyone.

After a few minutes of letting me stew in my anger, Facundo circled back, and I breathed a sigh of relief. When he pulled up beside me, he no longer looked annoyed.

"Can we please never do this again?" he asked. His voice was gentle — not a demand, but a request.

"This will be the last time," I agreed.

If, every time I rode, all I felt was pain and exhaustion, I didn't want to do it anymore. I felt resigned. Riding was no longer my happy place. Facundo slid his bike in front and slowed his pace to meet mine. When we caught up to Rose, she slipped in behind me, and the three of us silently made our way back to the finish line.

On the drive home, I was quiet. The ride and witnessing the car accident had taken a physical and emotional toll on me. Facundo didn't break the silence. Aimlessly watching the trees whizz by, I realized the absolute ridiculousness of my decision not to get the ICD. It was ludicrous. All the sports that I loved no longer provided any pleasure, only pain. Yet I was still trying to do all of those things, pushing myself through the pain with fingers crossed that I would live to see another day. Why did I think exercise was worth losing my life?

Facundo had already proven to me that my heart disease wasn't going to scare him away. He would support any decision I made. So how could I ask him to be my personal rescuer as well? What if my heart had stopped today, and he couldn't revive me? I asked myself what was worse: having a hockey puck sticking out of my chest, or constantly worrying that this could be my last day alive?

I turned to Facundo and announced, "I will call Dr. Laksman's office on Monday and book my ICD surgery."

He took his eyes off the road for just a moment, to see if I was serious, and then said, "Ok."

CHAPTER 13

FIRST STEP FORWARD

I still wasn't ecstatic about getting an ICD, but having made the decision did provide some relief. On the morning of November 21st, 2016, Facundo and I drove the short 1.5 kilometres from our apartment to St Paul's Hospital. On the drive, we chatted about spending Christmas with Rose and Benny in Palm Springs, and anything and everything except for the upcoming surgery.

We knew it would be a long day of waiting, so we brought my iPad with a Netflix series downloaded to keep us entertained. We walked the familiar corridors, took the elevator up to the fifth floor, and turned left to where a receptionist sat behind a glass partition which muffled her voice. It didn't matter. I knew the protocol now and could recite the answers she was looking for. Although I can appreciate the danger and risk of getting one patient confused with another, the constant repetition of questions every twenty minutes grated on my patience. "What is your name? What is your date of birth? Who is your emergency contact?"

A young nurse wearing scrubs and Crocs called my name, and as she led me into the cardiac ward, the routine began again. "What is your name? What is your date of birth?"

She cross-referenced the information, handed me two blue hospital gowns, and continued reciting her script. I crawled under the thin hospital sheet on the stiff upright bed and Facundo took his place in the chair to my left. I looked around the ward and noticed that I was the youngest patient by at least thirty years. Pushing the observation aside, I reminded myself that self-pity and comparisons were never helpful. Instead, I tried to keep myself distracted about why I was there by immersing myself in the imaginary lives on my iPad. I wanted to get the procedure over with as soon as possible, before I changed my mind. Ten minutes before my surgery, the nurse announced that my surgeon, Dr. Bashir, would be arriving to introduce himself and answer any questions we had before the surgery.

Dr. Bashir strode across the room with confidence and, after taking only one look at me, he asked, "Where would you like your device implanted?"

"What do you mean?" I asked.

The only information I had about implanted cardiac defibrillators (ICDs) was what I had gleaned from Google and the one-page handout that my client had given me after her father received his pacemaker. I had assumed that there were only two possible locations. The most common, and what I expected, was just below the left collar bone. The other location was around the left ribcage. Neither looked appealing, but I didn't realize I had a choice, nor did I know how to make that decision.

Dr. Bashir smiled and informed me that I not only had a choice but also a third option. The device could be hidden entirely by implanting it under the left breast, submammary.

"I have operated on yoga instructors, actors, and other women who would prefer to have their devices hidden for various reasons. Would this interest you?" Dr. Bashir asked.

I was both surprised and confused. Why hadn't someone told me of this option sooner? If I had known that I could hide the device, I would likely not have waited for an entire year. My mind was spinning with conflicting emotions.

Facundo finally spoke for me, "Kristina, isn't this what you wanted? Why aren't you saying anything?"

By some fantastic luck, chance, or karma, Dr. Bashir had offered a solution that absolved a few of my fears. I would have a backup in case my heart stopped and nobody, except Facundo, would see it. This was not the appropriate time to feel resentful.

Dr. Bashir warned me that the surgery was more invasive and required a longer recovery time than either of the other two locations, but I didn't care. I asked a few more questions about the logistics of the location and my physical limitations during the recovery phase and then agreed.

Dr. Bashir left the room and I never saw him again. I should have asked so many more questions. This little device would live inside my body for the remainder of my lifetime, and I had very little understanding of what that meant.

When I asked the nurse why I hadn't been informed of this third option before, she answered, "Most people with your condition arrive in the ER unconscious and wake up with the device already implanted. Or they don't wake up at all. They don't get a choice. You're one of the lucky ones."

That didn't answer my question, but it did shut me up.

It wouldn't be until the writing of this book that I learned more about why this placement is rare. The surgery had the potential for more complications, and in Vancouver there are very few surgeons capable or willing to do it. Every device requires a battery change every eight to ten years, so whenever my battery requires a replacement, I have to find another capable surgeon or hope that Dr. Bashir is still available. In addition, the majority of patients who require an ICD are typically older adults, less likely to care about the appearance of the device, and prefer a local, less-invasive procedure instead of general anesthesia. At the time of this writing, I had met only one other woman who had an ICD in the same location as mine.

***

This time when I awoke from surgery, I wasn't screaming, but I was talking. Feeling groggy, I had difficulty opening my eyes, but I heard Facundo chuckling beside my bed.

"What about rock climbing?" he asked, coaxing me to keep talking.

Slurring my words, I answered, "Ohhhh, you aren't that good. I's's— I's's a mushhh bedder climmer. You did … didn't make it da top … but I cud."

He was outright laughing now at my blatant, childish honesty. He had video recorded at least five minutes of me bragging about how great a rock climber I was and how much better I was than him.

My mouth felt so dry. I needed water. The nurse stuck a tongue depressor in my mouth and declared that I wasn't ready for water yet, but that he could give me some ice chips. With my brutal honesty and humour still in check, I didn't skip a beat and let out a sarcastic, "Whoopee, ice chips!"

He did not find my antics amusing. Nor did I get any ice chips. Instead, the nurse rolled his eyes and turned on his heel back to the nursing station.

A few moments later another nurse returned and helped me into a sitting position. She instructed me to walk around the ward, as the increased blood flow would help wear off the anesthetic. Feeling weak and off-balance, I leaned heavily on Facundo, and slowly we paced the ward, me in my paper slippers. My entire left side ached, and walking was the last thing I wanted to do, but I did want to go home.

I knew that the ICD was about the same diametre as a hockey puck and half the width. Still, it felt like it was the size of a small organic watermelon inside me. I shuffled up and down the cardiac ward with a watermelon under my breast, trying to comprehend how I had gone from being a competitive athlete to … whatever I was now, so quickly.

Finally, I passed the gag reflex test and was given the green light to go home. That first night at home, I crawled into bed and discovered that finding a comfortable sleeping position was tricky. Lying on my stomach was absolutely out of the question. I had stopped lying on my left side a few years ago as this position would trigger vertigo attacks, but now it also meant that I would be squishing the device.

My usual position on my right side hurt, as gravity pulled the ICD away from my chest, making it feel like it would pop out of my skin. The only option left was to lie on my back. Within minutes the pressure of the soft bed against my ribs felt like someone was driving their closed fist through my torso and directly up against my heart. My left arm went numb and my shoulder ached.

The only comfortable position was being propped up on three pillows, with a fourth pillow placed against my left ear so my head wouldn't drop to the side and set off the vertigo. This was my new sleeping position for the next several months until I had fully healed. Lying against my mountain of pillows, I felt some relief, knowing that I had a back-up should my heart stop, but ultimately I felt defeated. My life was never going to return to normal.

CHAPTER 14

NO SICK DAYS

The morning after my ICD implant, I stirred awake and raised my arms over my head in a big, good-morning stretch. The movement jolted me wide awake as a sharp pain shot through my left side. I had forgotten about the ICD. The pamphlet had warned me not to raise my arm over my head for several weeks so as not to dislodge the ICD or the leads into my heart. It needed time to build up scar tissue to protect it. I would definitely not be stretching like that again anytime soon.

I yanked my arms back down, and the shooting pain returned to the dull, heavy ache I remembered from the night before. My hand instinctively moved to my left breast, a habit that I would not be able to break for several years. Every morning, the first thing I did upon waking was to check if the implant was still there — a reality check.

I glanced over at the clock to see how long I had slept and noticed that I was lying in the exact upright position that I had carefully placed myself in 12 hours before. Behind the clock sat my remote monitoring system, the same system that I had previously used with the loop recorder. Every night, the monitor would upload the entire day's heart rhythms from my ICD via Bluetooth and send the information to a nursing station for monitoring. It was comforting to know someone was watching out for me, but at the same time I resented the intrusion into my life.

I could hear Facundo moving about the apartment but Naiya was still curled up beside me. Once she knew I was awake, she snuggled closer, nudging me with her nose, looking for attention. My thinking was still foggy from the anesthesia, but the realization of what I had done was crystal clear. A flash of fear gripped me. I started to question whether or not I had made the right decision. *I should be happy, shouldn't I? The ICD is almost completely hidden. Nobody but Facundo would ever know it was there. But what if he finds the device repulsive?*

Pushing away my insecurities, I decided that it was pointless to have regrets now. If I didn't want Facundo to be grossed out by my new internal hardware, then I had to pretend it was no big deal. If I didn't want my clients to worry that I was no longer qualified, I had to prove to them that neither my device nor my disease affected my ability to coach.

Facundo interrupted my thoughts when he came bounding into the bedroom, looking very much like an eager puppy. I could see that he was trying his best to be optimistic, wanting to cheer me up.

"You slept for 12 hours!" he exclaimed. "I'm so proud of you. You needed the rest, and you look so much better this morning."

I smiled, but inwardly cringed. *How depressing — that my greatest accomplishment is sleeping twice the amount of a normal adult.* I wished I didn't need so much sleep. I wished I could function on less.

Facundo bent down to hug me, but in anticipation of the pain from the ICD being squished, I instinctively flinched. He quickly recovered and changed course, giving me a quick kiss instead.

He helped me out of bed and to the closet where I surveyed my options. I hadn't thought this far. I wasn't allowed to raise my arm over my head but everything I owned — sports bras, tee shirts, hoodies — went over my head. He helped me get into one of my only real bras with a clasp at the back, an oversized tee shirt, and a sweater with a zipper at the front. I was grateful that he wouldn't be able to see my ICD or surgical scars for at least a week as we waited for the bandages to come off.

I was dreading that day, but decided not to think about it. At the moment Facundo was happy, taking some pleasure in caring for his patient. I didn't want to be the one to ruin that.

I smiled at his goofiness and lied, "Actually, I feel pretty good today. I don't think I need the painkillers anymore."

"No," he replied. "You need to stay ahead of the pain, especially if you want to get back to work tomorrow."

I had previously thought that the surgery was going to be a simple snip of the skin and placement of the device. When the surgery was changed last-minute to the more invasive submammary placement, it never crossed my mind that I may need to take more time to recover.

In the afternoon, Rose dropped by to check on me and brought a beautiful bouquet of flowers. I placed them beside the bouquet that my sister had sent from Calgary. I was touched, but the women's gestures scared me. I felt that they were making a bigger deal out of this than was necessary. When Rose left, Facundo encouraged me to go for a short walk to test my energy. But my mind proved to be stronger than my body. I managed to walk only two blocks to the beach before feeling completely spent. The thought of climbing back up the hill again was daunting and I sat on a bench to rest.

"Are you sure you'll be ready to go back to work tomorrow?" Facundo asked as I slowly, painstakingly walked the few blocks back to our apartment.

"I have to go back," I said.

Looking back now, I understand that I did not have to go back to work so soon. Financially, I could afford to take a few days off, and my clients would have been sympathetic and understanding. However, my belief at that time was that taking time off was lazy and irresponsible. My goal as a personal trainer was to teach by example, which included consistency and commitment. I placed my own mental and physical health second to my business and relied on my false belief that I could force my body to do anything I asked it to. Having an ICD inserted and being in a bit of pain wasn't a good enough reason to stay home.

But I had one problem. I wasn't allowed to lift anything over ten pounds for at least six weeks. I had warned my clients of this, but I had forgotten about my 6 a.m. circuit class. There was no way I could set up all that equipment for the class by myself. Instead of cancelling, Facundo agreed to be my assistant.

***

At 5 a.m., Facundo jumped out of bed in one shot at the first sound of the alarm. I resented his ability to be fully awake, alert, and happy within seconds of waking from the deepest of sleeps. It had been years since I felt that amount of enthusiasm, bounding out of bed, excited to greet the day. Since being diagnosed, I felt like I was in a constant state of lethargy. I felt old and damaged.

He helped me out of bed and into the same bra and a new tee shirt. *I'll have to get more practical bras,* I thought.

Facundo took Naiya out for her morning walk while I sat down at the kitchen table with a large glass of water and swallowed the pain killers, beta-blockers, and vitamins one by one. I forced myself to eat some dry toast and drank my coffee slowly, trying to clear the cobwebs from my head. At least I wasn't suffering from a vertigo attack.

As a precaution after the ICD placement, patients aren't allowed to drive for six weeks, so Facundo drove. As we entered the gym, we were greeted by the receptionist, Sarah.

"Welcome back! How are you feeling?" she asked.

"Great!" I lied.

For the next 20 minutes, I walked through the gym while Facundo trailed behind me, picking up the equipment I needed. We set up the exercise stations just in time and started the class at 6 a.m. sharp. Although my entire left side felt bruised and sore, it felt good to focus on something besides my problems. I walked around the room, giving advice, adjusting form, telling clients to add or remove weight.

At the end of class, the group helped clean up the equipment and chatted with Facundo for a few minutes before he drove home. I stayed for two more hours and trained two more clients. For just a little while, I forgot that I was a heart patient.

By 9 a.m. I had finished work for the day. It had only been three hours, and I was exhausted. I walked home and crawled back into bed. At the time, I chastised myself for not being stronger.

If I could go back in time, I would order my old self to stay home and allow myself more time to recover. I wish I had given myself permission to do nothing but read all day while my body healed. But knowing the type of person I was then, I likely wouldn't have listened.

CHAPTER 15

BRAS AND MARATHONS

My priorities had shifted from planning for the future to simply getting through the day. So when I awoke from my nap, instead of building programs or advertising classes, I decided that my most urgent problem was my lack of appropriate support bras. The ICD hurt anytime my left breast moved and all of my support bras required me to raise my arms over my head to get them on.

Instead of driving to the store, I decided that walking would be the most efficient use of time as it would double as exercise for Naiya, save time finding parking downtown, and allow me to get some exercise as well. And so this was how, two days after surgery, I found myself walking downtown to go shopping at Victoria's Secret.

Before anyone could tell me that dogs weren't allowed in the store, I marched down the escalator, past all the pretty lacy things, to the sports section in the farthest corner of the store. Out of the corner of my eye, I could see a young woman making a beeline for me, eager to make a sale. She was way too perky and smelled like vanilla, which made me nauseous.

"Would you like to try those on?" she chirped.

I barely looked at her. My chest, still wrapped in bandages, ached considerably after the 45-minute walk. The painkillers were wearing off.

"No," I growled, "I know my size."

She wasn't easily discouraged. "Did you know that most women wear the wrong size bra and have been for most of their lives? Would you like me to measure you?"

I had already found the sports bras with a clasp in the front. I chose two in black. Any bit of patience that I had been desperately clinging to had worn thin.

"No. Thank you," I answered. "I know my size. I don't need you to measure me."

"Can I at least give your dog a treat?" she asked.

"No," I said for the third time. "I'm in a hurry. We need to go."

In the new environment, Naiya pulled hard at her leash, wanting to say hello to everyone. With only one arm to hold her back, I was having difficulty controlling her and I couldn't risk dislodging my device if she lunged and jumped for treats. I made my way back up the escalator and paid for the bras.

As I left the store, I thought that I should have been kinder. But then quickly pushed any thoughts of the Victoria's Secret employee aside as I moved on to my next problem. My client and good friend, Dr. Ali Zentner, had invited me to travel to Honolulu with her to walk a marathon. Ali specialized in obesity medicine and used the Honolulu Marathon as a training goal to help motivate her patients and demonstrate what was possible. Along with her staff and thirty of her patients, my friend Cheryl and I had committed to the event.

It was still only two days post-surgery, but I wondered if two weeks was enough time to heal. At the time of registering for the event and booking my flights, I hadn't known I would be getting an ICD two weeks prior, but either way, nobody had told me that having the surgery prevented me from completing the walk. And although it seems like an insane idea now, that was par for the course of my life back then.

Before my diagnosis, I never would have questioned my ability to walk a marathon. I had raced Ironman, marathons, and long distances in the mountains, so I didn't think walking for 42 kilometres on a flat road would be that difficult. I imagined that I could post a photo at the finish line with the caption, "16 days after ICD surgery, I walked the Honolulu Marathon!"

I thought, *If I want to be an outlier and not let this heart disease beat me, isn't the marathon the perfect way to demonstrate this? Isn't that the type of inspiration I should be providing my clients?*

My ego desperately wanted to do it, but my body didn't want to be an inspiration to anyone. All my body wanted to do was find a way to stop the never-ending pain and exhaustion.

***

On day three after surgery, I got out of bed at 4 a.m. I ripped the tags off one of my new bras and gently placed it around my rib cage, careful not to put any pressure on the ICD. Since I wasn't permitted to drive, I decided to walk to and from work at the gym, which would also help me train for the marathon. The distance was short, only 2.5 kilometres. But that morning, the effort made my breathing heavy and laboured. My expanding lungs pushed hard on my rib cage and into the restriction of my new bra.

By the time I arrived at the gym, I was sweating and felt like I was suffocating. I rushed to the women's change room, pulling off gloves, toque, and GORE-TEX jacket as I went. Having reached the privacy of the change room, I reached under my remaining layers and unsnapped the front clasp of my new bra. With the release of pressure, I felt instant relief and slumped down onto a bench, gulping in large lungfuls of air.

I stayed like this for a few minutes, giving myself some time to recover. I remembered what the Victoria's Secret employee had said. *"Most women wear the wrong size bra for their whole lives."*

Why had I been so mean to her? She was only doing her job, and, annoyingly, she had been right. It wasn't that I had been wearing the wrong bra size for most of my adult life, but having a hockey puck under my breast, bandages over that, and a bunch of swelling had likely altered my size.

I would have to exchange the bras. I hoped the same employee would be there so I could apologize for being so rude.

I removed the bra altogether now and threw it into my gym bag. Once my heart rate slowed back down and I felt better, I trapped the offending appendage against my body so that it would not jostle the device and cause any more pain. As I was already cradling my left arm across my chest, I didn't think anyone would notice that I was also cradling my left breast, especially through all my clothing layers.

I stood up and gave myself a quick pep talk in the mirror. I didn't want to bring my problems to the gym and dump them on my clients — they had enough of their own to deal with. I squared my shoulders and walked out into the bright, overhead, fluorescent lights and the sound of a booming rap artist telling his "girl" that he "loves her for her body." I tried my best to ignore the words of the song, the mirrors, and the never-ending quest for body perfection.

CHAPTER 16

STICKY CUPS OF GATORADE

On December 8th, 2016, I boarded a plane for Honolulu. Despite my forced optimism, I still hadn't recovered from the surgery. My left side throbbed. Over the past few weeks, I had obsessed about whether or not I should attempt the marathon, even as my body screamed, "NO!"

Throughout the pre-marathon dinner, my mind replayed a loop of the most common motivational quotes: "No pain no gain," "Mind over matter," "Just do it," and even my own business slogan, "Challenge yourself." When it comes to exercise, it is often the mind we need to convince. But that day nothing made an impact. I couldn't access that woman who embraced pain like a badge of honour.

I began thinking of myself in the third person. *Kristina had loved racing and was always up for a challenge. Where is she now? Why has she deserted me when I need her the most?*

On the morning of the marathon, I awoke at 3:30 and laced up my running shoes. The race started at 5 a.m. so the runners could finish before the sun got too hot. The walkers wouldn't be so lucky. Cheryl and I predicted we could walk the distance in just under 7.5 hours, finishing around 12:30 p.m.

The atmosphere at the starting line of most marathons is tense with anticipation. The athletes are subdued, focused on the task ahead and the inevitable pain they will have to endure. But far at the back, in the walking corrals of the Honolulu Marathon, the atmosphere was the complete opposite. It was a massive street party with music, lights, and fireworks. Many of the walkers were dressed in costumes; everyone was focused on nothing more than having a good time. Their enthusiasm was contagious, so when the gun went off I found myself being swept up in the excitement of the celebration and I briefly forgot about my pain.

But as the music faded behind us and the sun made its appearance, the adrenaline of the party had worn off. I falsely believed that, once I started the walk, my body would go into "race mode," doing whatever it took to cross the finish line in record time. That's what I always did. But at the 5-kilometre mark, my body was demanding that I quit, and I searched for a reason — any reason — why I needed to finish the event. I couldn't think of anything except that I wasn't a quitter. I visualized myself crossing the finish line, but the image didn't conjure any positive emotions. I knew there wouldn't be any feeling of accomplishment, nor would I post anything. It would be the same as when I finished the Tour de Whatcom;

my only emotion would be relief that it was over and a promise to never do it again.

I didn't need to walk for 42 kilometres to learn what I already knew. It was painstakingly clear that I didn't belong in a marathon, or any endurance event, as an athlete anymore. After failing at the Tour de Whatcom, this should have been obvious, but I needed to fail one more time before I fully believed it.

As most endurance events offer several distances for the participants to choose from, I decided that I wouldn't just walk off the course. I would quit at the 10-kilometre finish line. It was the same as stepping off the treadmill at 20 minutes instead of 19:52 — there was a slight feeling of accomplishment in finishing on an even number.

Cheryl didn't argue or try to change my mind. Instead, she gave me a big hug and said, "Don't worry about it. It's no big deal."

At the 10-kilometre turn off, I said goodbye to Cheryl and pushed my way through the throng of walkers to cross the finish line. I felt remorseful for bailing on my friend, leaving her to walk the next 32 kilometres alone, but still I forged ahead. I avoided the volunteers handing out sticky cups of Gatorade and finishers' medals. I had registered for the marathon, not the 10-kilometre distance, so I was technically a DNF (Did Not Finish) and didn't deserve a medal. This was my first ever DNF.

I unpinned my race bib from my tank top and dropped it into a garbage can. Walking back to the hotel, I tried to sort out why quitting the marathon had been such a difficult decision for me. I had participated in so many events; one more shouldn't have mattered. But it wasn't the race that I cared about. What bothered me was the knowledge that although I could still coach and be a spectator, I would never again compete against myself or others. Losing this part of my identity hurt more than any physical pain in a race ever did.

Moving in the opposite direction of the marathon, I scanned the participants' sweaty, eager faces. Walking parallel to the beach, with the sun still low at their backs, they were enjoying a light breeze, oblivious to the pain they would soon encounter. The marathon course would eventually lead them away from the ocean and into the mainland where the air would be stifling and there was no escaping the hot, burning, black tarmac. But that would be hours from now. And, for most of them, being involved in something this momentous was motivation enough to push through any blisters, cramping hamstrings, or fatigue to reach their goal.

I understood the feeling perfectly. I knew what drove an athlete to train for hours and hours, day after day, year after year, to shave mere minutes off their finishing times. I had spent almost my entire life as one of them. I had never questioned where my ambition and endless energy had come from because it had always been a part of who I was. But now that I had lost that part of me, I didn't know how to get it back.

Feeling despondent and sorry for myself, I pulled my baseball cap lower, hiding my eyes. Back at my hotel room, I closed the blinds, shutting out the ocean view, and cranked the air conditioning up to the maximum, drowning out the sounds of the marathon music and tourists having fun on vacation. I put on my pajamas again and crawled under the covers.

CHAPTER 17

A MATTER OF PERSPECTIVE

I returned from Honolulu at an all-time low. No amount of journalling, walking in the woods, or pep talks from Facundo could stop me from crying. Every day my confidence dipped lower as I questioned everything about my life, including my role as a coach and personal trainer. If I couldn't keep myself healthy, how could I help others?

I contacted the BCIAP and asked them if they could connect me with other athletes who had ARVC. I wanted to talk to someone who understood what I was going through and could hopefully provide some advice on how to move forward. They connected me with two women, Allison and Claire. Immediately, I emailed Allison, who lived in California, and set up a walking date with Claire in Vancouver.

Both of them had been diagnosed six to eight years prior, so it should have been encouraging for me to see how well they were coping. Allison had given birth to three children and started an online business. Claire was full of radiant energy, and working full time. Watching her bounce off to her spin class, I ached with envy.

By this point, I had fallen too far down the rabbit hole of depression to see anything beyond how extraordinary they were and how pathetic I was. I wasn't able to hear their words of encouragement, nor could I see their lives as proof that my life would get better. I needed more than another pep talk — I needed professional help.

I first started seeing James Stabler, a Cognitive Behaviour Therapist, during the spring of 2009 when my boyfriend at the time had asked me to go to couples therapy. I learned a lot about communication and, even though we eventually broke up, I continued therapy on my own. Whenever I hit a roadblock that I couldn't see my way through or around, I would go back to visit James and he would help me climb over it. Once the problem was resolved, I would take a break from therapy until the next catastrophe.

I contacted James and booked his next earliest appointment time. James worked out of his home, which was an old stone house tucked away and hidden from the street by thick, bushy evergreens and a black iron gate. On the day of my appointment, I arrived early, so I leaned my bike up against his house and sat on the front steps to wait. I had learned from past experience that no matter how many times I rang the doorbell or how hard it was raining, James would never answer the door until exactly the appointed time.

"Setting boundaries," is what he'd say.

At precisely 1 p.m., James opened the front door. He was wearing black dress pants, a white button-up shirt, a maroon tie, and polished black dress shoes. He greeted me as if I had just seen him last week, although it had been several years since our last session. He ushered me inside and led me into his office at the far corner of the house. The room had large windows with heavy, green drapes shutting out most of the light. I took my usual seat on the plush, black-leather couch, slipped off my running shoes, and sat cross-legged, leaning into the cushions to get comfortable. Directly opposite the couch was James' desk and a bookshelf stacked with books from floor to ceiling. Everything about this room made me feel like a child — vulnerable, but safe and protected.

James pulled his computer chair around to face me and, with his clipboard and pen ready, started our meeting with, "Ok, so what's the problem that brings you back this time?"

James was unlike any other therapist I had ever worked with. He didn't navel gaze, nor was he interested in listening to endless hours of complaining or self-reflection. He wanted only the Cole's notes of the problem and would then go about finding a solution. Throughout the session, if I made any attempts to deviate or sidestep from doing the necessary work, he would sharply reprimand me, reminding me often that he wasn't interested in working with clients who weren't ready to help themselves.

I took a deep breath and looked down at my notes. *Stay focused, Kristina.*

He didn't interrupt as I quickly gave him the point-form version of the past year. While I spoke, I watched his face, looking for a reaction, but his expression didn't change in the slightest. He didn't sympathize, look shocked, or say any words of encouragement or empathy. This slightly disappointed me. I felt that my story was pretty remarkable and deserved at least a sympathetic head bob or two.

When I finished, he simply asked, "So how can I help?"

I tried to make the most of my time in therapy and always came prepared with notes and goals for the sessions. So I shrugged off my disappointment and looked down at my list.

James continued to listen. When I was done again, he stood up and, without saying a word, walked over to his bookshelf. Quickly scanning the titles, he selected one and pulled it off the shelf. When he turned around, he looked like a little boy with a secret, and he was going to make me guess what it was.

He flipped through the pages and found what he was looking for within seconds. It consistently amazed me that he always knew which book he wanted, and even which page the information was on.

I recognized the book. It was the bible. My heart sank. Was he going to tell me that God had a plan for me or some other such panacea?

Instead of reading the passage, he photocopied it and presented it to me like a gift. He had highlighted only one sentence — from Ecclesiastes. It read, *"There is nothing better for men than to be happy and do good while they live."*

I was annoyed. I looked up in confusion, but James continued to sit patiently, waiting for me to come to my own conclusion. I had spent all of my childhood in private religious schools and every Sunday morning in a church pew. These were not good memories. I resented the hypocrisy of the organized religion I had been a part of.

"I don't get it," I growled, refusing to indulge him by making any sort of connection for him.

He was not perturbed. He smiled and said, "Your purpose in life is to simply live. It isn't necessary for you to live up to any sort of expectation from either yourself or the people around you. These are all fabrications of your mind and society. Your only job on this earth is to live and be happy."

"But I'm not happy," I said bluntly. "That's why I'm here."

I started to think that this was going to be a waste of time. *Nobody understands the pain I'm going through,* I thought.

When he still didn't offer me anything more, I asked, "How can I be happy if I can't exercise? Not only am I too exhausted to do my job well, but I can't do anything that I love anymore."

James still didn't respond, but I could see that he was thinking. He stood up again and walked back to the bookshelf. This time he didn't photocopy anything but handed me a book. The title read *You Are the Placebo,* by Dr. Joe Dispenza. I flipped the book over and read the back. Paraphrasing, it read, "A Chiropractor/triathlete was hit by a car while racing and broke his back. The doctors said he would never walk again without surgery. Refusing the surgery, he cured himself through meditation."

That small bit alone made me furious. I continued to look down at the book, pretending to read as I organized my thoughts. *How should I respond to this?*

With a large dose of sarcasm I asked, "So you're telling me that I can just heal myself?"

His smile did not fade but he admitted, "I know the story sounds a bit far fetched, but you need to get past that and read the book. Dr. Dispenza explains that all physical ailments come from the mind. We are the ones who make ourselves sick, and so we also have the capacity to heal ourselves. Your heart disease, or at least the manifestation of symptoms, is your body's way of expressing a repressed fear, anger, past experience, or belief that you are still holding onto."

My face flushed red and my heart raced wildly. *How does he have the nerve to sit in his comfy chair, in his comfy house, and tell me that I created my own heart disease?* I thought. But I said nothing. Instead I began to cry. James pushed the Kleenex box toward me, and I grabbed a fistful.

For the past year, I had worked hard at pretending that I had accepted my diagnosis and was making the best out of a bad situation. But in reality, it felt impossible to let go of my identity as an athlete. I couldn't see any positives arising from the ashes of my situation. I had loved my life — everything about it — and I did not want it to change. The tears kept coming.

As all the emotions of the past year came pouring out of me, I wanted to remain angry, but something had shifted. Even though I didn't believe that my mind had created my own genetic disease, I couldn't deny the truth in what James had said. With surprise, I realized that my anger had been replaced with a feeling of relief. *Can I really stop training for endless hours, day after day?* I thought. *Am I finally relieved of any pressure to perform or even look a certain way?*

I had always thought of my body as a machine — a machine that I had full control over. I could see now that this machine had been urging me to slow down for many years now. Instead of listening, I had dulled the pain with extra-strength Tylenol and had refused to listen to the multiple warnings, so my body had simply shut things down. A defective heart was the one ailment I couldn't ignore. Even if my disease was genetic, I could see how I had potentially played a big part in my illness.

But the feelings of enlightenment and relief were brief. The question still remained: if I wasn't an athlete, then who was I?

James uncrossed and recrossed his legs as I dove back into the box of Kleenex.

CHAPTER 18

WHAT IF THIS WORKS?

I left James' office with an appointment for the following week and the title of Dr. Dispenza's book. As soon as I got home, I bought the ebook and collapsed, exhausted, into bed. It was three o'clock in the afternoon and, with Naiya's warm body curled up against me, I fell asleep.

One hour later, propped up on my pillows, I began skimming through the first few chapters of *You Are the Placebo*. Dr. Dispenza's theory is that our thoughts have the power to heal the body. Although we can't change our DNA code, we can use the placebo effect to change the expression. Dispenza states that we can rewire our brains by vividly imagining what we want to happen. I wasn't sure how all of this actually worked, and I didn't believe that my heart disease could be healed through meditation, but I was desperate and willing to try anything. As I read, my face flushed with shame. I couldn't believe that I had come full circle.

In one of my past therapy sessions with James, around six years before I was diagnosed with heart disease, we had been working on anxiety and depression. He had sent me off with a homework assignment: whenever I felt negative emotions like anger, depression, anxiety, or loneliness, I could not bike, run, swim, weight train, or even call a friend. Instead of masking my feelings with exercise, I had to stop whatever I was doing and just sit with the pain. I had known even as he explained the assignment that I would never do it. I didn't know how to do nothing. What did that even mean? But one week after that session, when I had been feeling incredibly overwhelmed with anxiety, I figured I should at least attempt James' method.

I had sat on my couch, crossed my legs, and closed my eyes. Within seconds my thoughts slammed into me like an angry bull, bucking and kicking me from all sides. *I am a failure. I am a horrible trainer. I don't know what I am doing. I am going to be alone forever.* Each negative thought felt like a kick to the stomach. I opened my eyes, angry that James would ask me to attempt such a ridiculous exercise. I made up excuses as to why this assignment didn't apply to me. *What does James know about exercise anyways?* This assignment might be suitable for some people, but exercising was my career. I couldn't waste precious time doing nothing when I could be training. Besides, my clients expected me to be in shape. So by exercising, I wasn't avoiding anything, I was just doing my job.

It didn't take much to convince myself that James was wrong and "feeling my feelings" wouldn't help me. I leapt off the couch, pumped up my bike tires, and left the house for a four-hour ride. When I returned home, my body and mind were numb with exhaustion, and the voices in my head had receded into the background where I could no longer hear them.

Now, sitting on my bed with *You are the Placebo* open on my lap, I realized that I should have listened to James' advice and done the homework when I had been healthy. Now I was out of options and distractions. I could not run, bike, swim, ski, or hike my way to happiness.

According to Dr. Dispenza, we create our own illnesses when we don't listen to our body's cues. I had become an expert at ignoring physical pain, pushing through every illness and injury. I chastised myself for being so stubborn and decided to start meditating that day, right at that moment. I sat up straighter in bed, placed my hands loosely in my lap like we did in yoga, and closed my eyes.

Immediately, negative thoughts came rushing at me in rapid-fire succession and in no particular order. I relived past events and conversations where I had said the wrong things, and caught myself wandering off into dream-like states of make-believe — all of it negative. Annoyed, I opened my eyes, set my timer for ten minutes, and tried again. I started to take in big belly breaths, inhaling and exhaling slowly to give myself something to focus on. This worked for about eight seconds, and then I caught myself planning tomorrow — what time I would wake up and which clients' programs I still needed to work on.

I opened one eye and peeked at the clock; only 4 minutes had passed. How could the act of sitting and focusing only on your breath be so hard? What was I missing?

On *The Moth*, they advertised an app called *Headspace*, which taught meditation. I picked up my phone and downloaded the free version, which included ten 10-minute meditations. Each meditation started with a cute 30-second cartoon explaining what you would work on during that session. I found the instructions helpful and they gave me something to focus on. I also enjoyed listening to Andy's calm, non-judgemental voice. Whenever I would beat myself up for getting distracted, I heard Andy say, "*Every time we get distracted is a lesson on how to start again.*"

On the eleventh day, I bought a one-year subscription. I imagined that, while my body was doing nothing, inside me was a busy factory with new neural pathways being created in the allotted 10 minutes.

One of the first lessons of meditation is to not have any expectations. This concept was foreign to me. I had a goal for everything I did in life. I didn't understand how it was possible to commit yourself to something without having expectations, so I ignored that part of the instructions. I scheduled my meditation sessions like a training program. Each week I lengthened the time by a few minutes and then began sitting twice a day, hoping to fast-track my healing and cure my heart disease.

A month later, during one of my meditation sessions, the cartoon instructed me to label my thoughts, then tap them with a feather to release them. It felt good to be in control of my thoughts, even if it was for only a few seconds. I was enjoying the process until I was hit with a thought that I couldn't tap with a feather, and my eyes popped open in fear.

What if this works?!

I ripped off my headphones, disconnecting from Andy's voice.

What if this actually works? What would I do if my heart disease was gone?

Instead of a rush of excitement and relief, I felt a sense of dread. My stomach and chest began to tighten, my breathing became shallow and rapid, and I could feel my pulse racing. It hit me that if my heart was healed, I would feel compelled to return to my old life, training intensely and working all hours of the day. I had started meditating with the goal of healing my heart, but now I realized that my heart wasn't actually the real problem. The problem was my mind and the expectations I had placed upon myself, driving me to excel. And why? I didn't even know. What I did know was that I wasn't mentally strong enough yet to resist working and training myself into the ground until some other part of my body failed

I started laughing at myself. I had been meditating for an entire month and thought nothing was happening. Without realizing it, my perspective had been shifting. It was finally apparent what my family and friends had been trying to tell me for most of my life. *"Kristina, there is more to life than fitness and exercise."*

I realized that the pain I was experiencing was the withdrawal period of not exercising. I needed to remain sick long enough in order to find peace and joy without using exercise to get it. Like an addict quitting cold turkey, I had to endure the suffering before I would feel good again.

Meditation was training for the mind. Similar to training the body, meditation requires repeated effort over a long period before noticeable changes occur. Understanding that I didn't have to do anything more than allow my mind and body time to heal, my stomach relaxed, and my pulse returned to its slow, steady crawl.

I continued to meditate every day, but no longer with the goal of healing my heart. My goal (yes, I still had expectations when I shouldn't have) was to learn how to find contentment in just being alive. Throughout that week, whenever I felt overwhelmed, I repeated the bible verse James had shared with me: "*My only job is to live and be happy.*" That one sentence was so simple, yet it relieved me of all the pressure I had put on myself. For now, I didn't need to be anybody or do anything more than just live. That was enough.

CHAPTER 19

WEDDING BELLS

After several months of meditating daily, my drive to exercise had done a complete 180. Now, if I was to engage in any physical activity, it had to meet a minimum of two of the following criteria: easy, fun, social, energizing, and outside in nature. But above all, it had to include my dog Naiya. I only had so much energy and she demanded a lot of it.

Ever since I had started my quest to become an all-around athlete as a teenager, I had pushed myself to extreme limits to grow and improve. I learned that if I wanted anything in life, I had to make it happen for myself. That drive and determination helped me build a successful coaching business and win several medals in the amateur field. But living with heart disease required a new set of skills and a different type of mental strength. I decided to work just as hard at healing as I had at everything else I had success with. I replaced my motto, "You can always do more," with "Simplify and do less." Healing became my new priority.

I became strategic about how much stress I took on each day and tried to plan for more recovery time. Stress didn't just pertain to sports and exercise. Stressing about updating my website, or having a fight with Facundo, took just as much energy as a workout. Recognizing that I had minimal energy resources, I permitted myself to nap whenever I could and was often in bed before 8 p.m. I still walked Naiya every day and exercised when I felt well, but I stopped striving to maintain an athleticism that was out of reach.

Within a year, I went from exercising over 14 hours a week to maybe 4 hours a week at most. At that time, I didn't count walking as exercise. This huge reduction in energy expenditure meant I also had to reconsider my diet which, up until that point, was dictated by what I thought an athlete should eat. Typically, my weight rarely fluctuated more than five or six pounds, but now the scale was beginning to tip too far in the wrong direction. I was acutely aware that everything that went into my mouth couldn't be burned off with a four-hour bike ride.

For years I counselled clients on how to lose weight and train for events, but my research focused more on athletic performance and less on overall health. I was now clearly aware that just because I had been physically fit, that did not mean I was healthy. And so began my new obsession with nutrition. I spent months researching the latest information and misinformation on nutrition, health and wellness, supplements, diets, and lifestyle choices. I bought audiobooks and listened while I walked Naiya, did laundry, washed the dishes, cooked, and drove. As soon as I finished one book, I would start another.

It took time to filter through what I believed was the truth and what I thought would work best for me. Many authors and experts contradicted each other, which explained why there was so much confusion about food. I was embarrassed to learn that some of the advice I used to preach had been debunked as outright lies made either by scientists in an attempt to further their careers, or by large corporations trying to sell more products.

Although the science of eating healthy is pretty straightforward, it becomes complicated when you bring in the human element. I thought about my clients, their diets, and the advice I had given them for the past 16 years. With so many factors playing into how each person digests, stores, and uses food for energy, it was impossible to believe that any single nutrition plan could work for everyone, especially when you factor in hormones, genetics, timing, environment, stress, culture, willpower, and individuals' history around food and dieting.

I went to my Kits Energy website and removed "nutrition counselling" from my list of services. Teaching an athlete what to eat before, during, and after an event was simple. Designing a food plan that encompassed and supported the health and wellness of each individual and their specific needs, while also taking into consideration the psychological damage of past trauma around food, was way beyond my scope of expertise.

Case in point, even with the knowledge that I had, since I had stopped exercising I had disregarded the nutrition plan I had followed for years. Eating healthy had always been an easy choice for me, as I knew it would result in a better performance. And yet, I had begun using food and alcohol as a replacement for that euphoric feeling I used to get from exercise.

On the one hand, I was terrified that I would gain weight without exercising; on the other hand, I wasn't doing anything to prevent that from happening. I was self-sabotaging my success in maintaining a healthy weight and healing my heart. Once I recognized what I was doing, and that the problem was something I had control over, I decided to make some changes. If I wanted to be an outlier to this disease, I had to start acting like one.

When helping clients, the first nutrition advice I gave — no matter the goal — was to reduce simple sugars, alcohol, and processed foods. This advice was universal; every diet and expert agreed on it. But following a restricted diet conflicted with my new motto of keeping my life as simple and easy as possible. I wanted to create healthy eating habits I could maintain and enjoy for the rest of my life. So I didn't eliminate any individual foods or count calories, and I definitely didn't analyze my daily macronutrients. Instead, I committed to making better food choices, more often than not.

In my quest to maintain a healthy weight and heal my heart, my friend Dr. Leslie Wicholas introduced me to an anti-inflammatory diet and helped me reframe my mindset around food. Leslie was an athlete, avid cyclist, and psychiatrist. In her practice, she designed a program which incorporated an anti-inflammatory diet to help her patients overcome or manage their symptoms of depression and chronic pain. Leslie believed that it wasn't enough to just avoid foods that harmed the body. Eating adequate amounts of specific vitamins, minerals, and foods with anti-inflammatory properties was vital. I also learned the importance of ingesting healthy bacteria to support good gut health and she gave me my first taste of kimchi and kombucha. I learned to like fermented foods and began to crave the hot spice of kimchi. I started brewing kombucha at home and replaced my glass of wine with a glass of healthy bacteria. My diet now includes a wide variety of nutrient-dense anti-inflammatory foods every day.

Like most athletes, I loved goals and had felt lost without something to work towards. With my new eating plan in place, I set a goal to lose the ten pounds I had gained since I stopped training. Since it had taken me almost a year to gain the weight, I gave myself ten months to lose it and chose September 16th, 2017 — our wedding date — as my goal. Yes, I did say wedding date. On May 21st, 2016, on Whidbey Island, Facundo had proposed.

Every bride wants to look her best on her wedding day, and I was no exception. Our wedding was a tangible, measurable goal that kept me focused on future possibilities instead of what I had lost. Losing the weight I had gained was the physical goal, but what I ultimately desired was to walk down the aisle feeling self-confident and happy in my skin again. I wanted to bring my best self — however that looked — into my marriage and our future together.

CHAPTER 20

GETTING CURIOUS

Even though I felt exhausted most of the time, my brain was still wired to want exercise. The urge was as strong as my desire to eat and drink. It was never an option for me to do nothing. If I couldn't do endurance sports anymore, I had to find other activities to fill the gap in my life. In addition, my relationship with Facundo had been built on training and exercising together. Without exercise, we needed to find other common interests. So we started our search for new sports and activities. I felt like a child, experimenting to see what I liked and which sports my heart could tolerate.

Facundo was one of the most accomplished athletes I knew. He could pick up any sport and, in a short time, he would excel at it. In 2015, he dedicated only three months to train for his first ever marathon, the BMO Vancouver Marathon. He finished in 32nd place overall, with a time of 2:47:56. This qualified him for the Boston Marathon the following year where he finished in 113th place, with a time of 2:38:30.

Justifiably, I was worried that Facundo would get bored waiting for me, but he insisted that my speed wasn't important. He enjoyed spending time with me, and the fact that he had to go at half his speed didn't matter. The only time he lost his patience was when I got frustrated with myself for not adapting to something as quickly as I thought I should. I was hard on myself. When my body didn't perform as it used to, I would sulk. But Facundo wouldn't permit me to ruin our day by having a pity party for myself and didn't tolerate it for long.

The first sport we attempted was indoor climbing. We booked a two-hour lesson at a climbing gym called Cliffhanger in East Vancouver. If I climbed slowly and didn't get overly nervous about the height of the wall, I found that I could keep my heart rate under control and have enough energy for about six climbs. After our lesson, we each bought shoes, a harness, and a chalk bag. The following week we returned, and I would have stayed until my fingers bled if Facundo hadn't insisted we stop.

Next was downhill skiing. When I lived in Whistler, I skied or snowboarded almost every day. But since moving to Vancouver almost 10 years ago, I rarely made the trek to the mountains. Facundo had never skied before, so we figured his lack of experience would help balance out my lack of cardiovascular endurance. We bought equipment from Craigslist and stuck to the green and blue runs. It was another success. If I went slow and took frequent breaks, I could ski for about four or five hours.

I loved the snow, and so, the next time we went to Whistler, we brought our skate skis. Skate skiing was another sport that I had introduced to Facundo, and I was excited to be back on the trails again. But the elation didn't last long. The moment I hit the first small hill, my heart raced out of control and I had to stop to catch my breath. I felt dizzy and faint and was nervous that my defibrillator would shock me. Facundo instructed me to ski slower, but the overall effort was too much and I had to turn back. Sadly, skate skiing was out.

Although I enjoyed the new sports, it took a long time for my body to recover after any athletic activity. Exercise was no longer a healthy way for me to relax, which meant I needed to find more sedentary hobbies. In addition, I wanted to find something that I could own for myself and reclaim my independence.

Serendipitously, during the fall of 2015, I had spontaneously registered for an eight-week mixed-media adult art class at a small studio called The ArtWay. Ironically, my first class coincided with my first cardiologist appointment, when the plumber told me I would be a fantastic candidate for a heart transplant. After the initial eight week class was over, I had signed up for the next class, and the next.

During that extremely turbulent year, the art class became my escape and the one thing I looked forward to each week. For three hours every Thursday morning, I allowed myself to get lost in exploring and learning. Much to my surprise, I discovered that creating art gave me a similar feeling as when

I raced and trained; nothing else mattered except what I was doing at that moment. Not only did I love the process, but I was proud of my work.

During that period of my journey, every day was a struggle, so Facundo was relieved to see that I had found something I was excited about. He encouraged me to keep going by challenging me to replicate a 34-inch-by-34-inch painting that we had admired at HomeSense. It was a simple painting of a single moose on a white background — nothing complicated. Although I had only been taking classes for a few weeks, he knew how much I loved working towards a goal and I took him up on the challenge. I became so obsessed with the project that the moose took on its own personality. I would stay late after class and often booked extra time on the weekends to work on my moose painting. Every week my sister, Jan, texted me, asking me how my moose was doing. I would send her photos and updates on my progress, keeping the final product a surprise for Facundo.

During the first week of November, right after the MRI and before my failed treadmill stress test, I completed my moose painting. I very carefully signed the bottom with a simple "Kristina" under his front right hoof. After waiting for the last coat of paint to dry, I gently picked up my painting and walked a few short blocks to my car. On the corner, a man passed me and did a double-take.

"Cool, I have that same painting. It's from HomeSense," he remarked.

I smiled broadly and nodded. "That's right."

Carefully, I placed the moose face up in the back seat of my Honda Fit and wrapped Naiya's blanket around the edges to protect it. I drove slowly and changed the gears gently so the painting wouldn't get knocked around or dented. Turning on the radio, I sang along with the country station. I brought the moose home and Facundo loved the painting, and even more so because I had found something that made me just as happy as exercise had. We hung it up on the wall in our office, opposite the mountain bikes. Every day, the painting was a reminder that my identity had so many more layers than just being an athlete.

As I stared at my moose, and the other paintings I had created over the past year, I realized that somewhere in my life, likely around the age of 15 when I had developed my strict training schedule, my definition of fun had lost all aspects of play. "Fun" to me was driving myself to sprint up a hill, pushing myself to the limit to win a race, or lifting more weight than I had the previous week. I didn't enjoy anything purely for "fun," in the frivolous sense of the word. Creating art taught me the importance of unstructured play for adults. I needed to add more play time to my life. I felt inspired to explore what other talents I might have hidden.

Most people described me as intense, focused, and sometimes intimidating. I was far from funny. But I had always wanted to be entertaining, free-spirited, and easy-going. Before the art class, I hadn't known that I could paint, so maybe I could learn to be funny? Before I talked myself out of it, I signed up for a weekend course titled "Introduction to Improv."

Before my first class, I dragged Facundo out to watch a few performances at the Improv Centre. I tried to imagine myself acting and reacting spontaneously on stage, but I couldn't picture it, and neither could he. Still, I didn't back out.

On the Saturday morning of the course, I was the first to arrive. I took a seat in the middle of the semi-circle formation and nervously tried to arrange my face to look friendly and less intimidating. My resting face is very similar to my race face and borders between angry and annoyed.

The remainder of the students filed in slowly, most of them late and looking like they had just woken up. While I waited, I tried not to grind my teeth with impatience at the other students' disregard for being punctual. Instead, I focused on the mantra I had ignored from meditation, "Have no expectations."

Within the first 20 minutes of the class, I found myself crawling on the ground, slithering like a snake, and then jumping up to do my best imitation of a lion. I felt ridiculous, and I loved it. I laughed so hard that weekend that I signed up for the next class. Unfortunately, my experience in the next class wasn't the same. The students were serious and the fun was gone. I realized I didn't like acting; I just wanted permission to be silly. I returned the next day to finish the course, but that was the end of my improv career.

In my past life, before my diagnosis, I would have considered the experience a failure. But with my new motto of having no expectations and choosing to only do things that I enjoyed, I felt not one iota of guilt about quitting, nor did it bother me. Without looking back, I moved on to my next idea: gardening.

I had killed every house plant, herb, or vegetable that had the misfortune of finding its way onto my third-story balcony. But I had always dreamed of growing my own vegetable garden. For a nominal fee of $15, I rented a small community-garden plot close to the gym, so I could attend to it before and after work. Over one summer, I didn't develop a green thumb, but I took great pride in being able to grow even a few vegetables, and the following year I rented two plots side by side.

I was enjoying my new life and exploring new parts of myself. I had stopped looking back with regret. I was once again focused on the possibilities of my future. Although I still didn't know what my life would look like going forward, I knew I would be ok.

It was during this experimental stage that I renewed a friendship with a past client, Walt Sutton. Although we had stayed in touch sporadically over the years, I hadn't heard from Walt since he moved to Seattle in 2014. Walt was an executive coach who spoke in front of thousands at conferences around the world, helping people grow and improve in business and, ultimately, life. During the time that I was his personal trainer, he often fed me tiny bits of advice that I savoured like organic 95% dark chocolate. Walt would leave the gym with a new training program and I would leave with a list of new authors to read and ideas to ponder. I enjoyed working with him and greatly missed our conversations.

When he emailed me in 2017, it came as a total surprise, and at just the right moment. Walt was in the process of retiring from his private coaching practice and was reaching out to see if I was interested in engaging in an ongoing conversation — a co-op, he called it. There were no schedules or time commitments. I could meet with him whenever was convenient for me and discuss anything that I wanted help with, all pro bono. Walt loved coaching and this was his way of remaining connected with the people who had positively influenced him. I was honoured and shocked that I had made it on his list and jumped at the opportunity.

Walt encouraged me to continue stretching myself to grow. He helped rebuild my self confidence and made me believe that, even though I couldn't see it, my future life was going to be even brighter than the one I had left behind.

Riding the momentum of being open to new experiences, I told Walt about my idea of writing a book. I have always loved writing and had published articles in the Vancouver Courier, on a cycling website called Women in Cycling, and in my own blogs and newsletters to clients. However, I had never tackled something as significant as a book. I wanted to write the story I was looking for when I felt my worst in this journey. I also needed to mentally process my experience, which I hoped I could accomplish by writing about it.

With some gentle insistence from Walt, I signed up for an online writing course called Memoir 101, and wrote my first (of many) "shitty first drafts" of chapter one of this book.

CHAPTER 21

MY NEW SUPER POWER

My new life and identity were beginning to take shape. Facundo and I found new sports we could share, and I enjoyed learning new activities that didn't involve exercise. And yet I still suffered from extreme envy of my friends and clients — anyone who was able to train at an intensity that was now beyond my capability. Every day was a reminder of what I had lost. Having decided that I wanted to remain in the fitness industry, this was one enormous hurdle I had to overcome.

My daily 20-minute meditations on *Headspace* had proven how powerful the practice could be in changing my perspective. I needed more of that. Hundreds of books have been written and classes taught on the subject worldwide, so I was convinced there had to be more to the practice than what the app could offer. Unsure where to start, I googled "meditation Vancouver." I chose an eight-week meditation course through Lightwork Meditation, because it was close to my apartment and fit my schedule. Nobody else registered, so I had a two-hour private lesson every Monday. The Lightwork method required enormous mental energy and focus, but I worked hard, never missed a class, and completed all my homework meditations. After each session, I felt a little less anger at the injustice of my diagnosis and, at times, could even put the feelings of envy on a low simmer. The style worked well for me, so when the eight weeks were finished, I signed up for level two and continued.

Halfway through level two, I noticed that it wasn't just my perspective that was shifting. I was becoming a different person, with different values and desires. On the weekends, when I drove Naiya to the woods and passed a group of cyclists, my heart no longer ached. While training clients at the gym, I didn't feel envious of their workouts or the fact that I would never exercise to the same intensity. In fact, not only was I not envious, but I actually preferred my life and the variety of outlets and interests I had recently discovered.

I was so excited with the shift that I began sharing my meditation experiences with my clients. I knew that if they could experience the same results, it would help them overcome many of their own hurdles and self-sabotage habits. They smiled politely at my enthusiasm, in the same way they did when I suggested replacing their glass of wine with a cup of tea. They were not convinced.

I felt an immense pushback on the topic of meditation in general. Only a select few who had practiced meditation for years were interested. I was overjoyed to find others to share my experiences with and learn from. But, at the same time,

I was slightly disappointed. I had high hopes that practicing meditation would result in a complete transformation where I would float around the world in a state of peace and contentment. But so far, none of the other meditators I had met seemed like they lived a blissful life, nor could I gather that they were calmer or more at peace with the world than anyone else. Several years later, I would read Dan Harris' *10% Happier* book on meditation, which I agree is a pretty accurate expectation.

Leslie Wicholas was the first person I could talk candidly with about meditation. She introduced me to Dr. Jon Kabat-Zinn's book, *Full Catastrophe Living*. Dr. Kabat-Zinn worked with patients coping with chronic pain who couldn't find relief using conventional methods. Through his eight-week course, he helped them where medication and other therapies had failed.

I was coming to understand that strengthening the mind was similar to strengthening the body. Both required hard work, dedication, consistency, and commitment — all qualities I had spent years developing. And like any health or wellness plan, there was no end goal. It was a commitment for life.

I liked this idea. But if I was committing to a lifetime of meditation, I wanted to be sure I was practicing the best method for me and doing it correctly. Although I enjoyed Lightwork, I was curious about other methods I had read about. My mentor, Walt Sutton, who was now my closest confidant and biggest supporter, suggested I try a Vipassana retreat. A "retreat" it is not. It is ten days of doing absolutely nothing except meditating in complete silence. My younger brother Jason had attended a retreat at the Vipassana Meditation Centre of BC and described it as one of the hardest things he had ever done. Ten days of sitting for hours at a time, doing nothing but following my breath, did sound exhausting, and I balked at the idea.

Interestingly, this was exactly the type of retreat my old self would have enjoyed, jumping at the opportunity to push my mind and body to new levels. But my new self flinched at the idea of inflicting more pain on myself. Every night I went to bed, having endured constant physical and emotional pain all day, only to wake up to do more of the same. I was at my complete capacity for pain.

But my curiosity was piqued by the technique of Vipassana. And as it happens, once you start thinking of something, you see it everywhere. While walking Naiya through the neighbourhood, I saw the same poster stapled onto light posts: an advertisement for a drop-in Buddhist meditation class at the Kadampa Meditation Centre. Again, the time worked with my schedule, and the class was within biking distance. I took that as a sign that I should attend.

The first class was led by Gen Kalsang Sanden, a Buddhist monk who looked very much the part. He dressed in orange robes with thick wool socks stuffed into well-used hiking boots, wore wire-rimmed glasses, and had a shaved head with a few weeks of stubble. Sanden sat in a plastic folding chair at the front of the room. About nine other students and I sat in a semi-circle around him. The class started with a 50-minute Dharma teaching which provided an idea or concept that we could focus on during the short 10-minute meditation that followed. The Buddhist ideas and concepts were liberating — so simple, and yet life-changing for me. Not wanting to miss anything, I wrote notes furiously throughout the class. I went back each week and replaced my Lightwork meditation practice with the Buddhist style, using my notes as a guide. After a few months, I could see the benefits of both styles and often interchanged the Buddhist style with the Lighwork energy practice, depending on my mood and how busy my mind was. Meditation felt like a new superpower, just like Dan Harris' book had said.

Once I made this discovery, I wondered, *Why aren't more people taking advantage of the power of meditation?* Again, I attempted to discuss the ideas I was learning in class with my clients. One morning at 6 a.m., while waiting for a client to warm up on the treadmill, I enthusiastically recounted my meditation experience from the previous evening. The focus had been on death — explicitly imagining our own deaths. The idea is that if you can experience how finite your life is (in the physical body), you can let go of daily worries that, ultimately, are not important in the grand scheme of your overall life. At the look of obvious horror clouding my client's face, I stopped talking mid-sentence and changed the subject. She seemed relieved and I reminded myself to never bring up meditation again unless someone asked.

Personal training, particularly coaching, is a delicate dance between two people. A good coach can assess when an athlete or client is ready to hear a new idea or move to the next level and will gently guide them forward. Sometimes I misread a client, offered too much information too soon, or pushed too hard when they weren't mentally ready to make a change. When that happened, the idea, the training method, and sometimes the entire relationship failed. Timing is critical. I learned quickly that convincing someone that they should adopt a habit — even a life-changing one — wasn't straightforward. I could never convince anyone to try meditation until they were ready.

I stopped talking about meditation but didn't give up on it. I would often sneak different forms into my client's workouts and wrote about the power of visualization in my newsletters. I used breathing techniques to help clients relax into a deeper stretch during a cool-down, and whenever a client arrived at the gym flustered or stressed, we started their session with a few minutes of box breathing to help them calm down. Most often, they left the session feeling better than when they arrived. Some even used the techniques to help them fall asleep or deal with stressful situations outside the gym. I never called it meditation, nor did I ask them to repeat the exercises independently, but I secretly hoped they would.

In all forms of fitness training, it is difficult to see gains from day-to-day activities. But then, one day, you surprise yourself. You run a split second faster, lift more weight than before, or bike up a hill more easily. Meditation is similar to physical training, just for the mind.

Every time I sat down to meditate, my belief systems were being rewired, little by little, day by day, week by week. Over time the feelings of depression and desperation were replaced with an overwhelming sense of gratitude for my life and the things that I could still accomplish. Instead of feeling stabs of envy whenever a bike whizzed by, I was grateful that I could still commute to work. Instead of feeling my heart rate rising in annoyance when a runner called, "On your left!" I was over the moon that I could still walk with my dog. I no longer sulked in self pity when Facundo tied up his shoelaces for a training run, nor did I dream wistfully of the times when I would spend the entire weekend riding my bike. I was content with my life. Meditation hadn't healed my heart, at least not yet, but it had changed my perspective, allowing me to see that I could have a fabulous life, even a better life, with heart disease.

Looking back, I realize how necessary the pain and suffering had been to my healing. Without the suffering, I would never have pushed myself to the extent I did to grow and change. When I was diagnosed, I thought I had to give up my identity as an athlete to move forward, but my journey has brought me full circle. No, I would never be competitive again, but that didn't mean I had to abandon my identity as an athlete. I will alway love and engage in sports, for as long as possible, but I no longer use exercise as a coping mechanism, nor is it my only source of happiness, entertainment, and identity.

I also feel that I became a better wife, friend, coach, and personal trainer in the process. I returned to my business with renewed energy, and greater understanding and empathy for the unique difficulties my clients faced, both physically and emotionally.

After six years of meditating, I would never claim to be a zen person. But whenever I get that itchy, agitated feeling that I used to calm with a run or bike ride, I know it is time to sit with my feelings. Meditation has become my coping mechanism.

CHAPTER 22

CHEATER

There was still one final fundamental problem that meditation or a change in perspective couldn't fix. It was clear that my heart arrhythmia would never permit me to ride fast enough to keep up with my riders and, although I had hired qualified coaches, I knew that if I wasn't cycling or participating in events, I would likely lose interest in coaching. Knowing this about myself, Facundo and I discussed the possibility of selling the cycling club or simply shutting it down. Since its inception in 2010, the club continued to steadily grow each year, until it reached a maximum capacity of 120 riders. We both enjoyed the work and the friends we had met through Kits Energy, so it would be a shame to let it go. In addition to disappointing the riders, it would also mean a big hit to my income.

Uncertain what to do and how I would pay my mortgage without coaching, I asked Walt for advice. At this point, Walt and I were meeting online at least once a month. He was empathetic, patient, and generous with his time. However, our conversations often circled back to the same problem. I thought that if I couldn't ride a bike, I needed to change careers or, at the very least, alter my business model. Walt wasn't convinced I had to do anything differently.

One day, when he must have known I was ready to hear it, he asked two fundamental questions that — to this day — I often fall back on: "What would happen if you didn't have an identity? Why do you need to label yourself as anything?"

I stammered, offering lame excuses in reply, but he just nodded and smiled. I could see that none of them held any ground. Having a label was comforting because it told me where I belonged. But if I didn't have a label, then I also didn't need to confine myself to the restrictions I had created under the labels of trainer, athlete, and coach. This was the same advice my therapist James had given me, which I used for my personal life but hadn't applied to my coaching role. I thought I needed to teach by example, but it finally clicked for me that not being able to ride didn't take away from my coaching expertise and knowledge.

When I really thought about it, now that I was no longer envious, I realized that coaching had become the closest thing to actually doing the sport myself. When I coached, I would often slip into a similar meditative state as when I exercised; nothing else mattered except for the athletes I was working with. The excitement I felt for them during a workout or event released a flood of endorphins without raising my heart rate. I enjoyed being an active participant in an athlete's success and introducing new riders into the world of cycling.

Once I removed the restrictions of what I thought a cycling coach should look like, it seemed apparent that I should continue coaching. Walt picked up on this excitement and suggested I find a way to be an active coach again.

Facundo and I discussed and researched the available options. Electric bikes were not yet popular in Canada and were just making their debut in Vancouver, so the pickings were slim. I decided on an EVO Fastway, mainly because it was the highest-end bike I could order through our sponsor store, Speed Theory. The black, 45-pound, hybrid bike would provide enough power to ride at 30 kilometres an hour on almost any gradient.

Unlike the purchase of all my other bikes, I wasn't thrilled with the idea of an electric bike. I didn't even test ride it before placing the order. It was a tool required for work, and that was all. When the bike arrived, Facundo had to convince me to ride it the few blocks home. I was embarrassed to be seen on it. I was afraid that the loud motor on the bike screamed "lazy" or — almost just as bad — "cheater." I was afraid that other cyclists would view me as a cheater for using a motor, which was precisely how I felt. I took the shortest route home and rode as fast as the motor would let me.

Facundo met me at home and helped me manoeuvre the bulky, 45-pound bike into our apartment, where I propped it up on its kickstand in the middle of the living room. Facundo laughed at the kickstand. Performance bikes do not have kickstands. We stood back and surveyed our new piece of furniture.

I knew what Facundo was going to say even before he said it. "Kristina, you have to sell a few bikes."

I didn't want to admit it, but I knew he was right. I owned five bikes, three of them collecting dust. I hadn't ridden my mountain bike since the day I was summoned to the emergency room after my 24-hour Holter monitor test in 2015. I also owned two road bikes, one for racing and one for bad weather, neither of which I had ridden since 2016 in the Tour de Whatcom ride. At that time, the only bike I was riding was the single-speed bike which I rode less than 5 kilometres for commuting to and from work.

I knew I would never race again, so it seemed logical that my race bike should be the first to go. I called it my race bike, but it was also the primary bike I used for training, coaching, and vacations. The bike was a 2007 white Cervelo R3 with so much history that it felt like an extension of my body. I had raced every triathlon, including Ironman, on that bike. I had flown with it to Hawaii to climb 10,000 feet to the top of Haleakala twice, and then to France to ride through the Pyrenees and the Alps with Rose. This bike had taken me on my first three dates with Facundo and helped build my coaching business. I had never planned on selling it. When the bike became too old, I would have demoted it to a winter bike, but I never imagined getting rid of it. But which was worse: having it collect dust in my apartment as a daily reminder that I would never ride it again, or selling it? It felt like I was deciding to euthanize my dog at the end of her life. I knew it was the right decision, but it hurt beyond belief.

I finally agreed to sell the Cervelo to a friend named Leah. Leah was just getting into the sport and would be joining my Introduction to Riding group that spring. When I dropped it off at Leah's work, my eyes were swollen red from crying. Seeing my bloated face, she almost started crying herself and offered to let me keep the bike. I was tempted to take her up on it, but holding onto a bike that I couldn't ride didn't make sense. Unable to speak, I shook my head no. I left the bike propped up against the wall in her office and ran back to my car. The pain of selling my race bike hurt for weeks, but once I tore off the bandaid, it made it easier to part with my mountain bike and winter bike.

***

On my first day coaching on my electric bike, I looked at my closet full of cycling kits and wondered what I should wear. In the past, I loved the ritual of putting on my sports gear. Everything had a specific purpose and being appropriately attired was the distinction between being a rider and being just someone riding a bike. But did riding an electric bike qualify me as a rider? I didn't think so. So if I wasn't a rider anymore, then what was I? I felt ridiculous wearing a complete spandex kit while riding a bike with a motor.

I asked Facundo what I should wear.

Without hesitation, he answered, "You wear your Kits Energy Cycling jersey and shorts, of course."

"But isn't that overkill? Won't I look silly?" I asked.

"Not at all. You're the coach and owner of the club. You should be wearing your club colours and signifying to your riders who you are. What's so confusing about that?"

That made sense to me. My kit was a uniform that I needed to wear for my job, never mind that it wasn't necessary to be aerodynamic.

I dressed in my Kits Energy Cycling kit and rolled my bike to the elevator. I hadn't even left the building and already I felt inadequate. I only lived on the third floor and had always carried my regular bikes up and down the stairs. The only time I took the elevator was when we moved furniture. The building was old, and the elevator took forever. I waited impatiently for the door to finally and painstakingly roll open. I squeezed the heavy bike into the small space, hoping that the ancient machine didn't get stuck between floors again and make me late.

I rode to the meeting point with butterflies in my stomach. I felt that I needed to explain why I was riding an electric bike and assure my riders that it would not detract from my ability to coach. I had planned a short, nonchalant speech, but when I saw Leah riding my Cervelo R3, a large lump gathered at the back of my throat. I could feel the tears threatening behind my eyes, and my speech turned into a strangled mess of random thoughts, mostly begging them to accept me. Afterward, my friend Ali pulled me aside and attempted to console me.

"Kristina, you don't need to explain anything to anyone."

I disagreed.

At the next workout, a rider who had missed my confusing confession speech the previous week demanded, "Why are you riding an electric bike? Isn't that cheating?"

My fear was verified.

Again, a few weeks later, during a coaching workout, I breezed past an older rider. He looked at me twice and then sprinted to get abreast of me again, just long enough to yell, "Cheater!"

I slowed my pace to match his and attempted to explain that I could die if I rode a regular bike.

He replied, "I'm 65 years old and I'm still riding."

While riding in the Ride Don't Hide charity event, a sponsored rider (this is what he called himself) pulled alongside me. For several minutes, he strongly voiced his opinion that I shouldn't be riding the event on an e-bike. Again, he said I was cheating. I pointed out that I was also an experienced rider, but I had a heart condition. Riding an electric bike was the only way I could participate. Since the event didn't provide timing chips and wasn't a race, I didn't see the problem. Ironically, I was riding to raise money for mental health while my own mental health was being challenged.

In each instance, I tried to come up with faster, more witty responses, but no matter what I said, I was still left feeling like a cheater.

When I complained to James, his response was, "So what? Why do you care what some stranger thinks of you?"

It bothered me because I agreed with them. Even though I knew the e-bike was necessary, and allowed me to continue coaching, I still felt like a cheater.

Through my therapy sessions, I learned that I didn't need to explain to anyone why I was riding an e-bike. I had to convince myself that it wasn't anything to be ashamed of. Knowing this didn't make me less self-conscious, but at least now I understood that I alone was responsible for my feelings and couldn't blame others for what they thought or said. By labelling the problem, James had planted the seed. Meditation allowed the seed to take root and flourish until, eventually, I could remove the stigma I had attached to riding an e-bike. It took an entire season for my ego to take a back seat.

It also helped that by 2018 electric bikes had become more popular, and everyone, including "cyclists," were taking advantage of electric power, especially for mountain biking. Ironically, in 2022, while I was writing this chapter and coaching my club on my electric bike, a triathlon coach called me out as a cheater in front of her entire riding group. Without any hint of embarrassment, I stopped and — smiling broadly at her and her group of riders — proudly replied, "Absolutely! I'm the coach. I can cheat all I want."

CHAPTER 23

WE DID IT!

In 2016, when Facundo had proposed on Whidbey Island, one of the first people I contacted was Steve King. For several decades, Steve had been the most famous and respected announcer of Ironman and many of the triathlon events held throughout BC. He had a knack for remembering details about every athlete, past races, and finishing times or placement. As you crossed the finish line, Steve King made those few seconds of glory more precious by briefly summarizing your racing season and sometimes adding a mention of family or friends supporting you. One summer, after racing the Peach Triathlon, I overheard another athlete gush about having Steve King officiate at her wedding. At the time, I had thought how cool that would be (if I were ever to get married).

Now I couldn't think of anyone more fitting to marry Facundo and me. We had met through the sport of triathlon, so although we had quit racing triathlon events, we had fond memories of those years. If I couldn't race anymore, at least I could have Steve King announce my name at my wedding. Steve agreed without hesitation and the date was set. We rented a large house on the West Bank of Penticton, BC overlooking Lake Okanagan and invited a small group of close friends and family for a full week of celebrations.

On September 16th, 2017, my father walked me down the aisle and into the arms of the man who had already proven to me that he would love me through sickness and in health. Neither of us knew how much my heart disease would affect our future, but with him beside me, I knew we could overcome anything. Since our engagement and my promise to myself — to bring my best self into this marriage — I hadn't entirely pulled the pieces of my life together. But I had created a blueprint that I knew I could work with. Yes, I did lose the 10 pounds I had gained, but more importantly, I felt comfortable and happy in my skin again.

After Facundo and I exchanged rings and kissed, I raised my arms in a celebratory salute, just as I would have after crossing the finish line. Facundo followed suit. That moment of pure jubilation was caught on camera and is one of my favourite photos. It was a triumphant and monumental moment in so many ways. We had done it!

But the story didn't end with Prince Charming whisking his princess away to their happily ever after. After the wedding celebrations, we said our goodbyes to our families and headed to the Vancouver airport for our honeymoon in Portugal, where I struggled. With the side effects of the beta-blockers making me feel like I always had the flu, and the excitement of the wedding wearing off, it took immense effort to ignore my chronic fatigue and continue to remain positive. In addition, while visiting Porto and the oldest parts of Lisbon, it didn't matter which path we chose: travelling from point A to point B always included several steep grades, both up and down again, just to go a few blocks. Facundo would often push me, literally, up the steep inclines, and still, I had to stop at the top to catch my breath, waiting for my heart rate to return to normal. Every night I collapsed into bed, completely exhausted.

When we returned from our honeymoon, I scheduled an appointment with Dr. Laksman to discuss other medications I could tolerate. Finally, after a year and a half of living in a beta-blocker fog, he took me off it and prescribed an anti-arrhythmic medication. Flecainide didn't affect my heart rate or blood pressure; it only treated the abnormal rhythms, which I was told would significantly reduce the adverse side effects.

Initially, I felt no difference. Then one day, while walking with Rose in the woods, I noticed I could actually climb a hill and talk simultaneously, without gasping for air. This was new! I felt my heart rate rising, adjusting to the increase in activity, but no negative effects. It felt wonderful to actually feel my heart beating again, pumping hard to keep up with my activity.

Over the next few months, I walked faster and further, pushing a little more each day to see what my heart could handle. When I could successfully hike up an incline without being out of breath or feeling fatigued, I added a small backpack with a ten-pound weight. I started dreaming about hiking through the mountains again and could see that, with some training, it might be possible.

Feeling confident that my heart could tolerate more intensity, I began experimenting with other activities, attempting sports I thought I would never do again. I switched from hatha yoga classes back to power classes. I skied all the way from Peak Chair to Creekside Gondola without stopping once and then went back up to do it again. In the spring, I rode my single-speed bike everywhere, challenging myself to ride every gradient without getting off to walk. As I had already sold my mountain bike, I borrowed Facundo's second one, and we tentatively rode a few trails on the North Shore. I was slow and had to stop often to let my heart slow down, but I was excited to be back on the trails. Although everything I did was at a much slower pace, I was able to do most of the activities I had missed for the past two years.

But the increase in exercise didn't come without some consequences. I still fatigued easily and often needed a few days to recover. After the more strenuous activities, I would experience a whole body ache, and my brain felt like it was full of cobwebs. The key was to do enough activity to enjoy an endorphin high, but not so much that I had to sleep for the next two days to recover. I was terrible at regulating myself, especially when I compared my fitness level to what I used to do. I always wanted to do more and often had to rely on Facundo to tell me when it was time to stop.

On my next visit to the BCIAP, I informed Dr. Laksman about my improvement and increased activity level. I didn't want to stop exercising, especially now that I had just gotten it back, but neither did I want to disregard his medical advice or speed up the progression of my disease. I wanted Dr. Laksman's permission and his guarantee that I wasn't damaging my heart.

Of course, he couldn't endorse my activity level or guarantee anything. Exercising went against all the medical advice and studies for my disease. But he promised that he would monitor me closely. If my condition worsened, I would have to re-evaluate my level of exercise. We both knew I was taking a risk but agreed that a patient's quality of life is sometimes worth a bit of risk.

As I write this, much has changed, especially since I was first diagnosed in 2016. New studies have emerged and, instead of restricting all activity, light exercise is recommended and encouraged. The rule I was told is "nothing too hard or too long, and definitely nothing hard *and* long." But "hard" and "long" are ambiguous terms that can be interpreted very differently from person to person, especially with athletes. There still aren't enough studies on patients and fewer still on athletes to know how much exercise is too much. It has been left up to me to decide, which I do day by day, week by week.

CHAPTER 24

INTO THE CANYON

In the summer of 2016, Facundo bought us a small camper van. Travelling in a van classified as a non-exercise activity we could share and also fit into my criteria of being easy, social, and including Naiya. Still, I wasn't so keen on the idea. I didn't enjoy camping and couldn't imagine what we would do all day in a van. Facundo found my lack of enthusiasm annoying but didn't let it deter him.

"That's fine. I'll go by myself," he'd said.

It was a blatant attempt at counter-psychology, and it worked. Begrudgingly, for my 41st birthday, I agreed to drive to the Oregon coast for the long weekend. And after only one trip, I fell in love with van life. We had all the comforts of home, including a king-size bed, toilet, hot water, three-burner gas stove, oven, and even air conditioning if we were plugged in. But what I loved most was the simplicity. Life was less complicated in the van, especially when Facundo made all the arrangements, drove, and took responsibility for all the messy parts, like emptying the black water tanks (a.k.a. the toilet). The fact that we could step outside our door right into nature was the icing on the cake.

Facundo and I worked long hours and we were often sleep-deprived. While travelling in the van, we never set a morning alarm and slept for 12 hours straight. After a few days of catching up on sleep, my sporadic vertigo attacks — which had plagued me since 2014 — became less frequent and I had more energy. We continued to venture further and planned longer trips throughout North America, exploring parks and beaches by mountain bike or by foot.

Naiya loved the van. Whenever we started packing for a trip, she'd jump in and refuse to get out. She was afraid we would leave without her, which we did, on this particular trip. In September of 2018, Facundo had organized a three-week hiking trip through three US national parks. Dogs are not permitted in the parks, and Naiya would never have survived the heat anyway, so this was one trip that we did without her.

Leaving on September 1st, 2018, we made our way to Bryce Canyon, Utah; continued on to the Grand Canyon; and then back up to Zion Canyon before driving home again. Hiking through the Grand Canyon had been a dream of mine. Now that I had just recently regained my ability to be more physically active again, I felt an urgency to do everything while I still had the chance.

In preparation, I had been hiking on the North Shore and in Whistler, but there wasn't much I could do to prepare for the elevation and extreme heat. In Bryce Canyon, the hiking trails started at 2,743 metres (9,000 feet). We walked through the most fantastic hoodoos, reminiscent of our trip hiking in Cappadocia, Turkey. The bright red and orange rock formations made for exciting scenery; however, we quickly discovered that the distances were deceiving. Starting the trails at the top of the canyon meant that the first half was almost strictly downhill on smooth non-technical paths, which made for an easy and fast pace. We only felt the full force of the heat and elevation when we turned around and started to exert effort on the climb back up. At that point, we had no choice but to keep going. There were no shortcuts, very few water stations, and no shade to escape from the unrelenting sun. Hiking in the desert can be brutal and even deadly if you aren't prepared.

However, Facundo and I were experienced hikers. We used the same training techniques while hiking as we did when we raced. We paced ourselves for the distance, constantly monitored our hydration and fatigue levels, and followed a strict refuelling schedule — eating every 45 minutes. Heat stroke and bonking are preventable, but we knew that even the most prepared and experienced hikers could run into trouble. Although I only carried a light pack, Facundo carried a full backpack with all of our emergency supplies — fire starter, portable shelter, warm clothing, water tablets, emergency food, and a small first aid kit — in case we got stuck and had to spend the night in the wild.

On each hike, we ventured further and tested my limits. Facundo monitored me closely. Whenever I got frustrated with my lack of cardiovascular fitness, he reminded me how far I had come since my diagnosis in 2016. He knew I was getting tired and that it was time to cut the hike short when I lost my temper or became irritated with the heat, flies, or other hikers.

We spent three days in Bryce Canyon before moving on. Driving to the Grand Canyon's south rim, we stopped only briefly to take photos of the more popular tourist attractions. Arriving late, we parked the van and went to sleep. The following day, the sun was already high when we stepped outside for our first view of the canyon. It wasn't the most beautiful view, but it was one of the most awe-inspiring. Standing on the edge was so remarkable that it conjured up the most conflicting feelings — intensely powerful and humbling at the same time.

Our first day in the Grand Canyon was scheduled as a rest day, so we spent the afternoon exploring and talking to the park rangers. We watched the information videos, read up on the hikes, and strolled along the rim, trying to take it all in. Facundo liked to tease me by placing his toes over the edge of the rim until I begged him to move back. It was a 1,829-metre (6,000-foot) vertical drop to the bottom. It made my stomach turn watching him get anywhere within a foot of the edge.

Throughout the park, numerous signs warned tourists of the dangers of hiking in the Grand Canyon. Specifically, the signs said to not attempt the hike from the rim to the Colorado River and back in one day, which was exactly what we wanted to do. Park rangers tried to scare us out of the idea by recounting the story of a woman — a doctor no less — who had attempted it the previous year and had died. They were not clear about the conditions that resulted in the woman's death, but it was a very effective warning. Although we were confident in our hiking capabilities, I wasn't so sure about my fitness level.

Hiking to the bottom and back would be a massive achievement for me, and I desperately wanted to complete it. But if my body failed me, the consequences could be fatal. What would Facundo do if my ICD went off while we were hiking? What if it went off prematurely? What if I got to the bottom and couldn't hike back out again? The story of the woman dying the previous year spooked me. And reading the warning signs that stated, "Hiking in the canyon is not recommended if you have a heart condition," didn't help either.

I wrestled with the idea for a few days, unsure if my fear was valid or if I was using my disease as an excuse. I didn't want to risk my life, but I also didn't want to live in fear.

The very fact that hiking to the bottom and back in one day had an element of risk to it made it tempting and exciting. It was then that I realized I hadn't lost that woman in me who loved a challenge and was up for anything. Although she had lain dormant for several years, she was still there. Now I could feel her poking me in the ribs, urging me to grab this opportunity. My motto of keeping my life simple and easy had been necessary when I needed to be kind to myself and allow my body time to heal. But I was stronger now, and my heart was more capable. I hadn't come this far just to become passive and let life pass me by. I accepted the challenge.

We decided we would attempt the hike on our second-last day in the canyon. Our plan was to start hiking at 4 a.m., giving us a few hours to walk in the coolness of the early morning and provide some buffer time. Facundo set two alarms — one for 3:15 a.m. and another for 3:30 — just in case we slept through the first one. Once everything was packed and we triple-checked that we hadn't missed anything, we crawled into bed, and immediately Facundo fell asleep.

I lay on my back and stared at the ceiling a few feet above my head. I was nervous, plagued by how the next day could go disastrously wrong. I tossed and turned, and for what felt like the twentieth time, I checked my watch. Midnight. Facundo snored softly beside me, oblivious to my fears. If he was awake, I knew he would reassure me that I would be fine. I trusted Facundo, and he wasn't often wrong, but what if this was one of those times?

I must have dozed off because when the alarm went off, I jumped up and almost hit my head on the low ceiling. I was wide awake, more awake than I had been in a long time. I was excited. Now that it was time to act, the idea didn't seem so scary anymore. We dressed quickly, grabbed the breakfast sandwiches we had made the night before, and stepped out of the van. The temperature was just above five degrees Celsius. I pulled on my winter coat, toque, and gloves. As we made our way to the bus stop where the bus would take us to the trailhead, I gazed up at the sky, lit up with stars. The weather forecast had been correct. It was going to be a clear day with no chance of rain.

On the bus, we were the only passengers. The driver seemed happy to have some company. He asked a steady stream of touristy questions, which Facundo answered for the two of us. I ignored the conversation. I wanted to remain focused on what I was about to do. The feeling of anticipation was similar to when I used to race. Although there wouldn't be any prizes and I wasn't competing with anyone, not even myself, I knew that at some point, the hike was going to hurt.

The driver dropped us off at the Bright Angels trailhead and then carried on with his day. In all of the scenarios of what could go wrong that day, I hadn't considered wild animals. But standing in the parking lot alone, in the dark, with nothing but our backpacks, I had images of coyotes and other wild animals that could attack a vulnerable human. I did not voice this fear to Facundo as I knew he would think that I was becoming hysterical.

We turned on our headlamps and, locating the start of the trail, cautiously began our descent. We moved slowly, aware that any misplaced step could mean a sheer drop to the bottom. Ahead of us were a few more headlights bobbing up and down, telling us that we weren't the only ones attempting the hike that morning.

Once we started moving, the butterflies in my stomach began to quiet, and I settled into what I expected would be a very long day. The trail was wide and worn smooth from millions of hikers and horses before us. It wasn't long before the sun began to rise. We watched the light play tricks, changing the colour of the rocks, as the sun made a path across the sky. Every 45 minutes, Facundo's alarm told us it was time to eat — 250 calories and at least one litre of water. By the second alarm, we had already peeled off all our winter layers. The temperature continued to climb until it reached well over 30 degrees Celsius. There wasn't a cloud in the sky and rarely a tree to shade the route.

After fuelling correctly, the next important aspect of endurance training is pacing. In any long-distance sport, everyone feels strong when they begin, and it is tempting to think you can maintain that pace for the entire event. But training stress accumulates deceptively slowly. If you aren't careful, eventually the body will get to a point where it won't be able to perform essential bodily functions. This is unfortunate and can sometimes be dangerous in a race, but when hiking in the desert or on a mountain, it can be deadly.

Starting the hike so early gave us a substantial buffer should anything go wrong and allowed us to take our time, stopping for photos. Even still, we surpassed Facundo's expectations and arrived at the Colorado River at 9:30 a.m. with lots of time to spare. I was relieved and ready to head back up again. But Facundo reasoned that it wouldn't take much more effort or time to hike to the famous Phantom Ranch resort, which was only 3 kilometres further along the river. Again I asked myself if this was an unnecessary risk, or if I was using my disease as an excuse not to experience life. I doubted I would get another chance to hike into the canyon anytime soon, or ever again, and decided that this was an opportunity I didn't want to miss.

On our way from the river to the ranch, I heard the familiar call, "On your left!" and jumped to my right. Turning around, I was expecting to see a mountain bike or maybe a horse, but instead it was three runners, light on their feet as they bounced from rock to rock. Each of them carried only a small hydration pack and nothing else. Wistfully, I watched them until they were out of sight and felt a familiar stab of envy.

Before my diagnosis, that could have been me. I could have run to the bottom and back up again.

The feeling lasted only briefly before I gave my head a shake. Last year I could barely walk up the small incline to my apartment, and now I was hiking the Grand Canyon! I had nothing to be jealous of.

I pushed the feelings aside and looked up. It was so far up to the rim of the canyon that it took my breath away. Being at the bottom gave me an entirely different feeling than standing at the top. At the top, I felt powerful and strong, but at the bottom, I realized how minuscule and insignificant I was in this vast world. It felt liberating to know that my little life wasn't really all that important. When I died, this canyon, the river, and these rocks would continue without me until the end of time. It reminded me that I shouldn't take my life so seriously and should enjoy every moment. I only had one life, one chance. I thought, *If only I could bottle up this feeling of gratitude for when I go back home.*

At the Phantom Ranch resort, we bought ice-cold cans of Coca-Cola and sat on a bench in the shade. We revelled in the feeling of being minuscule specks at the bottom of the enormous canyon. When we felt that we had stayed long enough, we left the safety of the resort and began retracing our steps. Returning to the river, Facundo wagered that, even with the additional hike to Phantom Ranch, we still had lots of time to spare. Again, he wanted to delay our ascent — to take a dip in the Colorado River. Swimming in the river was another thing the rangers had cautioned us about. The current was strong enough to create a massive canyon, so it could easily carry even a strong swimmer downstream, never to be seen again. The muddy water and the warnings were enough to deter me, but Facundo was determined. He was an extremely competent swimmer and didn't usually take dangerous risks, but I still worried and was grateful that he didn't venture too far. I snapped photos of Facundo swimming along the shore, and when he had swum long enough to say he'd done it, he climbed back out. He dried off, dressed in his sweaty clothes again, and we resumed our trek back to the top.

Having already taken numerous photos on the descent, we remained focused on our mission to climb to the top safely. We hiked at a steady pace, resting only briefly, either when my heart rate felt too high, or whenever we could take refuge in the few places that offered shade. When we crested the rim at 2:30 p.m., our finish was anticlimactic. No one screamed my name, hung a medal around my neck, or congratulated me on my achievement.

But I was beyond elated. We had hiked 30 kilometres and climbed 1,421 metres (4,662 feet) in 10 hours. For Facundo, hiking this distance, especially at my pace, wasn't a significant effort. But I had accomplished what I had once deemed impossible. Just two years prior, I thought I would never hike again, and now I had just hiked the Grand freakin' Canyon! I wanted to savour the moment and recognize it in some significant way. But except for a hug from Facundo and a few random high-fives from the other hikers, we didn't do anything special. It was not in either my or Facundo's personality to offer gratuitous compliments. We simply sat on the rim of the canyon for a long while, not saying anything at all. After the journey we had been through, not just that day but throughout the past two years, nothing more needed to be said. Recognizing and being present in the moment was the best and only way I could think of to celebrate.

When I was diagnosed with ARVC and told that I would never be able to exercise again, I worked harder than I had worked on anything else in my life to find new purpose and joy. Now that I was back to doing most of the things I loved, although at a much slower pace, I didn't want to forget those lessons. I knew how easy it would be to fall back into old habits.

Gazing into the vastness of the canyon, I tried to recapture the emotions I had felt while standing at the bottom. I wanted to imprint those feelings of freedom, gratitude, and insignificance into my subconscious. I didn't want to revert to my default mode, constantly pressuring myself to perform and work harder. I didn't want to lose sight of the most critical things: my health and my relationships.

CHAPTER 25

RETURN TO CYPRESS

In the Spring of 2019, I signed up for the Triple Crown for Heart, a charity ride raising money for the BC Children's Hospital heart unit. Combining my passion for cycling with raising money for a charity that meant so much to me felt like the perfect fit.

I hadn't attempted to climb Cypress again since that fateful day on August 16th, 2015, when I collapsed in the ditch. The 75-kilometre ride for the Triple Crown for Heart included climbing three mountains on the North Shore — Seymour, Grouse, and Cypress — for a total elevation of 2,300 metres. The finish line was at the top of Cypress Mountain.

Before my diagnosis, I never questioned whether or not I could cycle up any mountain; it was only a matter of how fast I could do it. But now the simple act of riding a bike without a motor assist was a big deal, let alone climbing a mountain. And although I had regained confidence in my physical abilities, I knew my limits. There was no way I would be able to ride up all three mountains. My goal was to complete the last quarter of the event, which included only Cypress Mountain.

By 2019, my heart arrhythmia had stabilized and I had significantly increased my activity level. Although I still coached on an electric bike, I had convinced myself I needed to add another bike to my small fleet, and bought an Argon Dark Matter. It was a beautiful gold-coloured gravel bike with wide, knobby tires and a gearing ratio that made climbing easier. This was precisely what I needed to ride up Cypress again without increasing my heart rate excessively. Although I no longer followed a training program, my time mountain biking with Facundo and riding my single-speed told me that I was physically ready for the challenge.

I decided that since I wasn't riding all three mountains, I would start my climb later in the morning and join the riders as they ascended their last mountain. Like all cycling events, once the participants crossed the finish line, they were rewarded with a party — music, draw prizes, and a barbecue lunch. I wanted to be there when everyone finished, so we could share in the celebration.

On the morning of July 20th, 2019, as all the other cyclists lined up at the Ron Andrews Community Centre in North Vancouver, I was still at home sleeping. When the gun went off at 8 a.m. and the riders made their way towards Seymour Mountain, I was eating breakfast. While they rode up and down Grouse Mountain and across North Vancouver, I packed up the car and drove with Facundo and Rose to the base of Cypress Mountain. In the past, knowing everyone was riding while I was doing nothing would have tormented me. I would have felt like I was wimping out and missing out. But I had none of those envious feelings now.

At 11 a.m., I parked the car and we unloaded the bikes from the bike rack. On the front of my bike, I pinned my "race" number — a cute red heart with the number 26 printed on the front and my emergency information on the back. Since I was starting my ride on the last mountain, I didn't even have a formal start line or a starting gun to tell me when to go.

I put on my cycling shoes, gloves, and helmet, and realized that never again would I suffer from pre-race jitters. Due to the health risk of raising my heart rate too high or for too long, I would never again test my limits or put myself in the physical pain I had long become accustomed to. Unlike when I had first been diagnosed, this thought wasn't negative. I no longer felt pressured to perform or live up to anyone's high standards for physical fitness — including my own. I could return to my teen years and enjoy the act of riding, just because it made me feel good.

Similar to my hike in the Grand Canyon, this ride was a tremendously meaningful moment for me. Riding without a motor assist signalled that I was physically strong again, but it also signified enormous personal growth. I had spent a year mourning the loss of exercise and had come to terms with this reality. So now that I had been given a second chance to participate in the sports I loved, I appreciated every opportunity and treasured every workout like it would be my last.

Rose and Facundo also understood the significance of this day and offered to ride with me as my escorts. I'm sure they were also a bit worried about me riding alone. With the two of them flanking me, I pushed off, clipped into my pedals, and began climbing. I no longer rode with a power meter, and I definitely didn't make any attempts to stay on anyone's wheel. I simply paced myself to finish the distance.

At almost midday, the sun was high in the sky, warming the pavement and the riders. There was barely any wind, making the conditions idyllic for a Saturday afternoon ride. We climbed and chatted; about what things, I don't exactly remember. I was too overwhelmed with the euphoric feeling of being back on my bike, climbing Cypress Mountain with my friends and clients. A client and former nurse, Jennifer Bibby, rode alongside us, taking photos as we climbed.

As my legs pushed the bike up the unrelenting 6-percent incline, I felt my heart respond appropriately, driving more oxygen into my muscles. My heart beat strong and steady in my chest and my ribs expanded to take in more oxygen. The feeling was delicious. Even so, I rode with some trepidation. Although I had a back-up this time, I didn't want to test the strength of my defibrillator and ruin the day.

During the climb, we passed other cyclists participating in the event who were completing the total distance. Some of them were from my club, and others were riders I didn't recognize. I encouraged all of them to keep going. By this point in their ride, they had been cycling non-stop for over three hours and were feeling fatigued, while I had just started and was feeling fresh. As I neared the 9-kilometre mark, I tried locating the exact place where I had laid myself and my bike in the ditch four years earlier. But, fortunately for me, there were no flowers, nor a cross, to mark the spot.

When we crossed the finish line, I realized I had forgotten to turn on my stopwatch. Facundo announced that we had finished the climb in just under one hour. Mentally, I noted that it was twenty minutes longer than I used to climb the same route. But my time was no longer relevant. The fact that I had made it to the top without incident — no shortness of breath, fatigue, chest pains, or feelings of passing out — was all that mattered. My body, and specifically my heart, hadn't disappointed me.

As more Kits Energy riders and friends crossed the line, I congratulated them on a fantastic achievement, and they did the same for me. Most of them knew about my journey and how I had struggled with my fitness, so they understood the day's significance. I snapped photos of the group, ate a burger, and listened to their stories. Some of them had ridden the event several times and had been trying for a personal best. Others were disappointed that they hadn't performed as they had expected. But everyone had a story of the moment when they had wanted to give up but didn't and persevered to the finish. I enjoyed listening to their stories, and could relate to each and every experience.

When Facundo, Rose, and I descended the mountain again, I rode at my own pace, taking in the view of the city as my bike floated me to the bottom, where we packed up and started the drive back home again.

AFTERWORD

At the start of 2020, COVID-19 was all anyone could talk about. One by one, I watched every country go into lockdown, and on March 17th, 2020, I finally understood what that meant. Like many others, my life and business came to an abrupt halt. As a non-essential service, the gym was forced to close. On that day I drove home in a daze, uncertain about anything. Like many people, I initially assumed the shutdown would be temporary.

Since there was nowhere to go and no commitments to keep, I was forced to rest. Every night I clocked a solid 12 hours of sleep. After a few weeks, I noticed that I no longer woke up with a headache and I could think more clearly. The vertigo had subsided and the daily exhaustion I had suffered from for almost a decade was substantially reduced. I hadn't felt this healthy for many years, nor had I realized that I still could. Even after all I had learned with my heart disease, it took a pandemic to show me that I still had so much more to learn about myself — specifically what it meant to truly take care of my health. I had known that sleep was vital for recovery and was also aware that I had been severely deprived of it, but without vastly reducing my income, I couldn't find a way to get enough rest.

This was a hot topic that Walt and I had discussed over the past year. Although I knew I needed to reduce my work hours, I was afraid to take the risk. The two hours before and after a nine-to-five work schedule were prime times for a personal trainer. I would be forfeiting a large portion of my income just to sleep. In addition, these were not just 10 hours a week that I would be giving up; these were 10 clients with whom I had developed strong relationships, some over 15 years. Choosing not to work during those early morning hours meant I would have to say goodbye to my friends.

However, when they announced an extension to the lockdown, I was forced to pivot and change. This period in my life was one of which I am most proud and I attribute much of my success to the lessons I learned in the year after my diagnosis. Within a few weeks, I adapted my personal training and coaching business to work virtually. By the time we were permitted to return to the gym, I had successfully transitioned 60% of my personal training business online. In the process, I also created a more balanced work/life schedule that was less stressful and gave me more time to rest and recover. Once I experienced firsthand how much better I could feel with more sleep, I promised myself I would continue to do whatever it took to guard my rest time.

For all of 2020 and well into 2021, I slept 10 to 12 hours every night. Although I lost precious productivity time, I no longer felt sick and was a much happier human, which in turn made me better at everything I did. Learning from this experience, I now adhere to stricter work/life boundaries.

Being diagnosed with heart disease greatly affected not just mine but also Facundo's life. If the roles had been reversed, I'm not confident I would have been as patient as he is. Facundo never complains about adjusting our activities or having to wait for me in any and every sport. When he sees me struggling, he now offers gratuitous compliments, yelling back loudly, "You are doing so great! You are amazing!"

I feel embarrassed, knowing that everyone can hear him and can see that no, I'm not doing amazing. In comparison to my fitness prior to my diagnosis, I'm actually doing terrible. But comparing myself with anyone, especially my past self, is never constructive. So I appreciate the motivation. His enthusiasm helps me remember that he is right, I am doing great! Nobody else on the trail knows how hard I have worked, and, likely, nobody is as grateful as I to be there.

Friends and clients frequently ask me if I am "better" now, to which I reply, "Yes and no. It's complicated." Yes, I have found a healthy way to exercise, but no, I am not "healed." Until they find a cure for ARVC, I will always suffer from heart disease and I will continue making compromises in my life to adjust to the progression of the disease.

Scrolling through my Strava or Instagram feeds, you'll see that I exercise daily, but nowhere close to the same level of intensity as I used to. Before my diagnosis, I pushed myself to improve, suffer, and win. Today, I exercise because I love to move my body and participate in activities that I enjoy, hopefully without further damaging my heart.

As difficult as it is for me, I don't follow a training schedule. My day-to-day life is already active, teaching online classes and coaching. If and when I do have time or energy to add an additional workout, the activity I choose depends on how much stress I am under and what areas I feel need rebalancing. I may use the time to build muscle strength or do the complete opposite and meditate to strengthen my mind. Sometimes I take a nap. The key is to be aware of what my body is asking for and remain flexible enough to follow through with the correct action.

Deciding how to spend my time is easy when I am rested and grounded. Other times, I catch myself overworking or over-exercising in an attempt to keep up with the imaginary ghosts of productivity. When I'm focused on a goal, it can take weeks to recognize that I have fallen back into old bad habits. Either Facundo will notice and alert me, or my body will tell me. Many old symptoms will return — headache, vertigo, nausea, and constant fatigue. Writing this book has been a daily reminder of what I value and how I wish to live my life.

Since we bought the camper van, Facundo and I have attempted to break the cycle of "constantly being productive" by taking an extended vacation every autumn. After a busy summer of coaching, we have made it our tradition to spend three weeks exploring parks and trails throughout North America, on bike or on foot. Disconnecting from email, social media, and almost all forms of communication allows us to recentre ourselves and refocus on what we value most. We return feeling rejuvenated and recommitted to our goal of living our best lives, each in our own way.

Living with ARVC is a daily reminder to take nothing in life for granted. I understand that my heart disease can progress slowly or that my heart can deteriorate suddenly without warning. Every year, when I visit Dr. Laksman, I am nervous, afraid that he will tell me that I can no longer hike up mountains or explore the trails on my bike. There are no guarantees that what I am doing today, I will be able to do tomorrow. So, whenever I ride my bike, hike a mountain, or even go for a walk, I take more pleasure in it than I did in any of my past race wins. Stressing about my speed, time, or watts is a luxury I can no longer afford.

Being diagnosed with ARVC forced me to re-evaluate everything. It was an excruciating process. But living through this struggle has been one of my life's greatest gifts. My diagnosis allowed me to rewrite my story, but becoming the person I truly want to be is an ever-changing, evolving process. Now I know that no matter what happens, I am, and always will be, an athlete at heart.

BIBLIOGRAPHY

Dispenza, Joe. *You Are the Placebo.* Carlsbad, California: Hay House Inc., 2014.

Harris, Dan. *10% Happier.* Dey Street Books, 2014.

Kabat-Zinn, Jon. *Full Catastrophe Living.* New York City, New York: Bantam Books, 2013.

ACKNOWLEDGEMENTS

I always wanted to have a great story to tell. Unfortunately, the most interesting ones require the protagonist to suffer greatly, before they can learn from their experience to become a better version of themselves. I never imagined how hard that process was, until I went through it myself.

There are several people who played an integral part in my journey. The first is my husband, Facundo, who never settles on self-pity as a solution to any problem. I can't thank him enough for his patience as I struggled to accept my diagnosis. He gave me the space and time to find my own solutions, which also included the five years where I dedicated most of my free time to writing this book. Although there were times when I may have wanted a softer and gentler approach, his push to continue moving forward was exactly what I needed.

Although it may not be customary to thank a dog, I can't downplay the role Naiya has played in my recovery and throughout my life. Emotionally, when I have nothing left to give, I can always rely on Naiya's unconditional and undemanding love to keep me going. On many days, she is often the only one I see or talk to all day. As my constant shadow, simply taking care of her gave me purpose when I felt I had none.

Although these women only get a few mentions in the book, I am forever grateful to Rose Cifelli and Cheryl Shkurhan, who were my patient walking companions. Every week, they listened to my rants without judgment. Also, Ali Zentner, who knew then, more than I did, how big a deal this diagnosis was, and celebrated my ICD operation with a girls' tea party and trip to Hawaii. Only in retrospect can I appreciate how scared I really was at that time.

Throughout my journey and the writing of this book, I feel that the people I needed to meet arrived at just the right times. The first was Walt Sutton, who reached out when I was in the middle of my struggle. Our monthly co-op conversations kept me focused on the person that he always knew I could be. He remains my biggest cheerleader and one of my closest confidants.

Leslie Wicholas, who I met by pure chance while riding my bike to Iona one day, helped alter the trajectory of my recovery, twice. I always leave our conversations with new information to research and ideas to ponder. Our friendship is a good reminder of how our words have an enormous effect on others.

I have known Elese Sullivan for many years, but it wasn't until I was looking for beta readers that I discovered she had been a writer in her past life. Elese spent countless hours combing through multiple drafts, offering an equal measure of advice and compliments, which greatly boosted my writing ego. But it was Elese's questions that I valued the most. She never skimmed my work, and when I fell short, she always called me on it. Her gentle approach of simultaneously recognizing work well done, while also challenging me to go deeper, is a trait that I hope to emulate with my own clients.

Another opportune meeting, at just the right time, was with my editor, Elise Volkman. Elise possesses the same talent of balancing criticism with praise and I consider myself extremely fortunate to have found her. With the aid of her podcast, *The Tea Grannies*, and multiple follow-up emails, Elise was a constant resource while I muddled through the self-publishing process.

Thank you to my beta readers, Walt Sutton, Margie Scherk, Ruby Mawira, Jack Grushcow, Rita Bangma, and Jan Rintoul for asking tough questions and providing honest feedback. A few had the unfortunate luck of editing some of my earliest work, while others benefited from more polished versions. But no matter which stage I was at, each offered a unique perspective which helped organize my thoughts and get them on the page with more clarity.

Dr. Martin Hosking, Connie Ens, Jackie Forman, and Serena Kutcher were also so kind to donate their time and offer their own personal and professional edits to the story, as well as ensuring that I didn't use any incorrect medical terms. Their generosity was beyond what I had ever expected, especially since a few of them only know me as a heart patient.

Lastly, I want to express my extreme gratitude to all the medical personnel and specialists who have helped me, specifically Dr. Bregman, Dr. Teal, Dr. Laksman, James Stabler, and Dr. Bashir. Most of them will remain in my life for a very long time and I can't thank them enough for all their efforts in helping me live my best life.

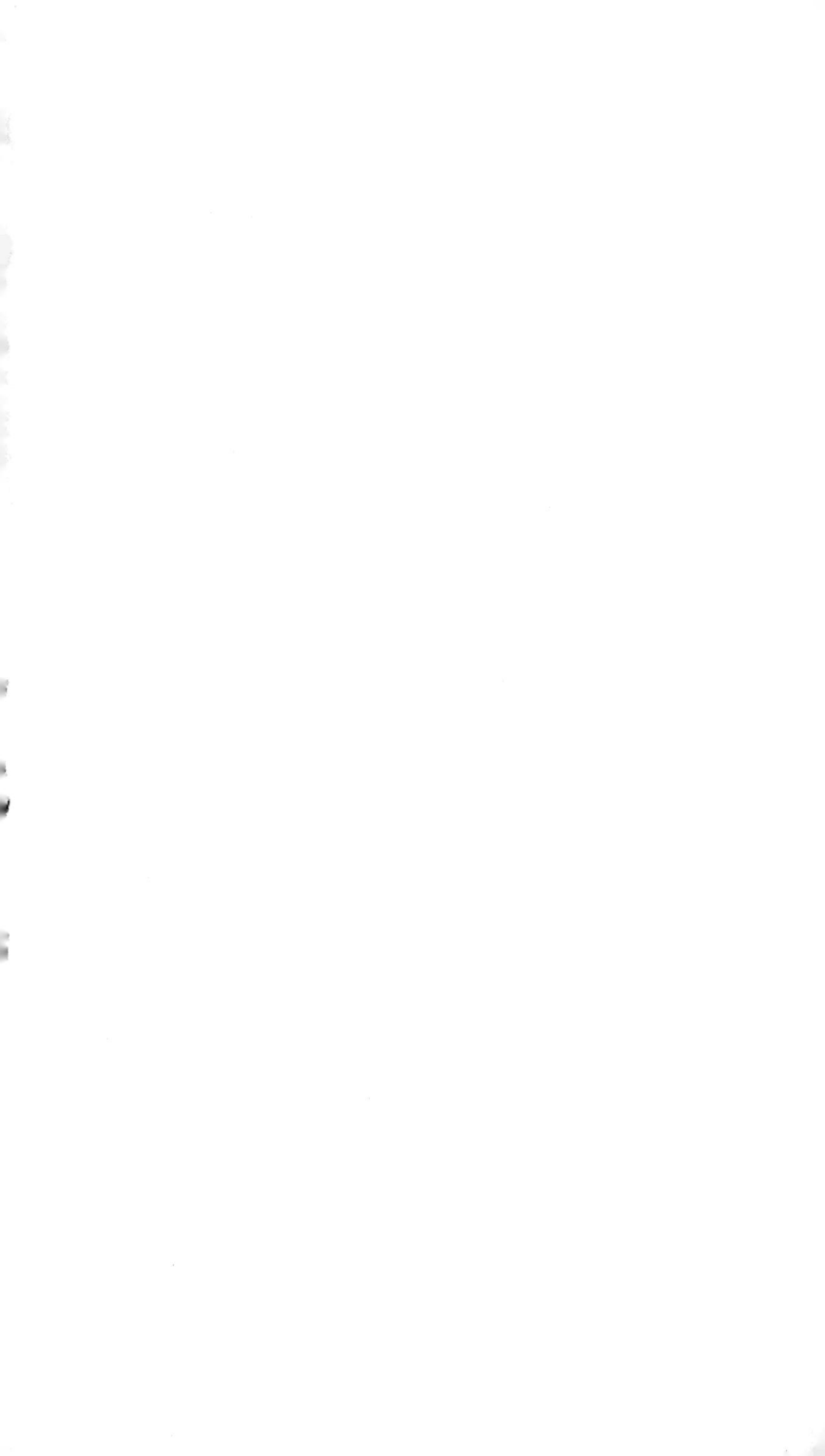

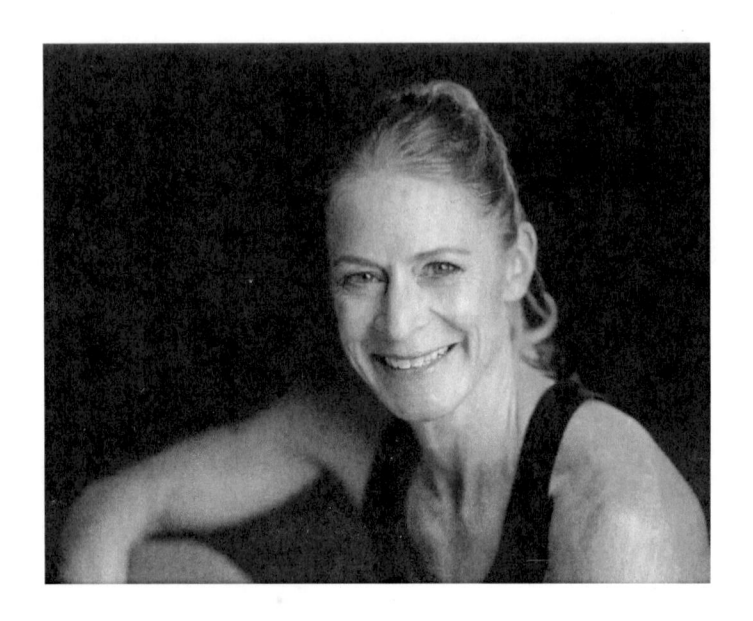

Kristina Bangma is a personal trainer, endurance coach, writer, entrepreneur, all-around athlete, and an ex-competitive runner, cyclist, and triathlete. She is the founder and owner of Kits Energy Training Inc. Kristina lives in Vancouver, BC with her husband, Facundo, and her dog, Naiya. *Athlete at Heart* is her first book.

   https://kristinabangma.com
   Facebook: @kristinabangma
   Instagram: @kristinabangma